Y0-AAQ-677

To my husband, Wes, for his patience, love, and words of encouragement to see this project to completion.
To my daughter, Emiley, for keeping her fingers crossed.
To my nursing colleagues, who have inspired my personal and professional growth.
To my parents for the gift of the belief that you can do anything you put your mind to.

Beverley Tipsord-Klinkhammer

To my family, Caesar, Tricia, Domenic, and Laura, for their love, support, and encouragement, and . . .
To my angels, my mother who taught me the art of caring and the unlimited rewards of education and hard work, and to my brother, Tim, who taught me the importance of family and unconditional acceptance of all people.
I know you are there.

Colleen P. Andreoni

In addition, we wish to acknowledge the MacNeal Health Sciences Resource Center for the help given.

Beverley Tipsord-Klinkhammer
Colleen P. Andreoni

Preface

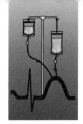

Emergency nurses recognize the need to stay current on a variety of procedures, medications, disease signs and symptoms, and trauma treatment in the ever-changing field of emergency nursing. While textbooks on the specialty of emergency nursing are available and widely read, it is impossible to carry a large textbook in a pocket.

Quick Reference for Emergency Nurses will provide the reader with 25 useful, concise chapters geared to the practicing emergency nurse. The information will be helpful for the novice emergency nurse as well as the most seasoned professional.

This ready reference is meant to be informative and easy to use. This is a useful tool that will serve as an adjunct to the knowledge obtained from a class and a lengthy textbook. It is not meant to be a primary source of detailed information. Rather, it is a primary resource for common to not-so-common emergency nursing procedures, medications, treatments, and *pearls.*

Beverley Tipsord-Klinkhammer
Colleen P. Andreoni

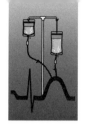

Reviewers

Irene Borze, RN, MS, CEN
Faculty, Nursing Division
Gateway Community College
Tempe, Arizona

Linda V. Hackley, RN, MS, CEN
Swedish Medical Center
Englewood, Colorado

Roselyn Holloway, RN, MSN
Methodist Hospital School of Nursing
Lubbock, Texas

Linell Jones, RN, BSN, CEN, CCRN
Lakewood, Washington

Sandra B. Knight, RN, BS, CEN
Naples, Healthcare System
Naples, Florida

Denise Marie LeBlanc, RN, BScn
Humber College
Toronto, Canada

Chris Miller, RN, MS, CEN
Director, Emergency Services
Swedish Medical Center
Englewood, Colorado
1995 President, Colorado Emergency Nurse
  Association
Denver, Colorado

Debra Siela, RN, MN, RRT, CCRN
Ball State University School of Nursing
Muncie, Indiana

Jeanne Whalen, RN, BSN, CEN
Emergency Department
Carolinas Medical Center
Charlotte, North Carolina

Contents

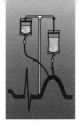

DRUG NOTICE

Emergency Nursing is an ever-changing field. Standard safety precautions must be followed, but as new research and clinical experience broaden our knowledge, changes in treatment and drug therapy become necessary or appropriate. The editors of this work have carefully checked the generic and trade drug names and verified drug dosages to ensure that the dosage information in this work is accurate and in accord with the standards accepted at the time of publication. Readers are advised, however, to check the product information currently provided by the manufacturer of each drug to be administered to be certain that changes have not been made in the recommended dose or in the contraindications for administration. This is of particular importance in regard to new or infrequently used drugs. It is the responsibility of the treating physician, relying on experience and knowledge of the patient, to determine dosages and the best treatment for the patient. The editors cannot be responsible for misuse or misapplication of the material in this work.

THE PUBLISHER

Chapter 1
Abdominal Emergencies

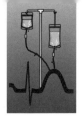

AUSCULTATION OF BOWEL SOUNDS

- Emergency Department (ED) assessment: Auscultate for two minutes (see Table 1–1)
- Descriptors
  - Quiet, loud, occasional gurgles
  - Fine, loud tinkles
  - Absent (after two-minute auscultation)

Table 1–1. Auscultation of Bowel Sounds

Description	Possible Cause
Hyperactive	Diarrhea Early obstruction
Hypoactive, absent	Paralytic ileus Peritoneal irritation
High-pitched tinkling sounds	Intestinal fluid and air under tension in dilated bowel
High-pitched rushing sounds with abdominal cramping	Intestinal obstruction

- Bowel sounds audible in the chest indicative of ruptured diaphragm
- Ausculation of abdominal bruit or hum not normal

COMMON ABDOMINAL SIGNS
(see Table 1–2)

REBOUND TENDERNESS

- Often painful: perform at end of abdominal assessment
- May be local or general
- Sign of peritoneal irritation
- Procedure
  - Slowly press fingertips near area of reported discomfort, applying deep pressure (depress 4–5 cm)
  - Quickly withdraw fingers, release pressure

Table 1–2. Common Abdominal Signs

Sign	Indication
Coopernail	Ecchymosis on scrotum or labia suggests fractured pelvis
Cullen's sign	Purplish color around umbilicus suggests blood collection in abdomen from fractured pancreas or ruptured ectopic pregnancy
Kehr's sign	Referred pain to left shoulder and left upper quadrant suggests splenic rupture or irritation of diaphragm from blood, bile, and fecal material
Turner's sign	Bluish color on flank suggests blood collection in abdomen from fractured pancreas

- Positive rebound tenderness produces pain as the abdominal tissue springs back after deep pressure is applied and quickly released.

SEAT BELT SYNDROME

- Improper use of seat belt may cause abdominal injury. Problems include
  - Lap belt without shoulder harness
  - Shoulder harness without lap belt
  - Improper placement of lap belt
- Mechanisms of injury are associated with car crash
  - Deceleration forces
  - Compression of abdomen by seat belt
  - Increased intra-abdominal pressure
  - Increased pressure within hollow organs
  - Rupture, laceration, or herniation of abdominal organs
  - Shearing stresses
  - Tissue tearing, organ transection, or vertebral injury

HEPATITIS

- Hepatitis A (HAV), "infectious hepatitis"
  - Fecal-oral transmission
  - Incubation: 10–50 days
  - Symptoms: fever, anorexia, nausea, vomiting, diarrhea
  - Associated with crowded living conditions, often seen in children
- Hepatitis B (HBV), "serum hepatitis"
  - Sexual and parenteral transmission
  - Incubation: 40–180 days
  - Symptoms: nausea, right-upper-quadrant pain, malaise, anorexia, urticaria, low-grade fever

- Hepatitis C (HCV), "post-transfusion non-A, non-B hepatitis"
  - Parenteral transmission
  - Incubation: 15–160 days
  - Usually asymptomatic: chronic liver disease may persist for years.

CHOLECYSTITIS

- Hepatoiminodiacetic (HIDA) scan
  - A functional radioisotope test
  - Failure to see gallbladder suggests cystic duct obstruction
- Ultrasound of gallbladder: detects cystic duct stones, gallbladder wall thickening, and pericholecystic fluid
- Murphy's sign
  - Instruct supine patient to take a deep breath as the right upper quadrant or gallbladder is deeply palpated.
  - A positive sign is right upper quadrant or midepigastric sharp pain, arrested inspiration. Pain may radiate to shoulders and back.
  - A positive response suggests cholecystitis. Differentiate between biliary colic and cholecystitis (see Table 1–3).
- Interventions include
  - Parenteral narcotics: Opiates (morphine) are contraindicated because they cause biliary duct spasms.
  - Position for comfort
  - IV hydration
  - Antiemetics
  - Decompression of GI tract

APPENDICITIS

- Common cause of an acute abdomen
- Classic symptoms:

Table 1–3. Differentiation Between Cholecystitis and Biliary Colic

Biliary Colic	Cholecystitis
Obstruction of cystic duct	Obstruction of cystic duct
Short duration (<6 hr)	Longer duration
WBC normal	Leukocytosis
Afebrile	Fever
Often discharged to home	Patient is usually admitted
Pain occurs 3–6 hr after large meal	Pain begins as colicky and progresses to constant discomfort
Nausea, vomiting, dyspepsia	
Nursing interventions include administration of analgesics	

- Pain originates in periumbilical area and moves to the right lower quadrant
- Preferred position is supine with legs flexed
- Classic presentation is not as common in young children and elderly.
- Retrocecal appendix may present with right flank pain.
- Positive iliopsoas test
  - Right-lower-quadrant pain with passive extension of the hip or with moderate resistance over the thigh as patient flexes right hip
  - Suggests inflamed or perforated appendix
- McBurney's point: area of localized pain and rebound tenderness between umbilicus and right iliac crest
- Associated symptoms
  - Anorexia

- Nausea, vomiting
- Fever
- Malaise
- Diarrhea or constipation
- Elevated leukocyte count
- Increasing pain with movement
- Ultrasound may assist with diagnosis

"GI COCKTAIL" (SHAMROCK SHAKE, GRASSHOPPER)

- Terminology depends on facility.
- Provide temporary symptomatic relief of minor esophageal and gastric irritation
- Common preparations contain
  - 30 mL antacids
  - 10 mL viscous xylocaine
  - 10 mL Donnatal elixir (belladonna alkaloids, atropine sulfate, hyoscyamine sulfate, phenobarbital, and scopolamine hydrobromide) or 20 mg dicyclomine (Bentyl)

Bibliography

Budassi Sheehy S: Mosby's Manual of Emergency Care, 3rd ed. St. Louis, Mosby–Year Book, Co. 1990.

Budassi-Sheehy S, Marvin J, LeDuc Jemmerson C: Manual of Clinical Trauma Care: The First Hour. St. Louis, Mosby–Year Book, 1989.

Emergency Nurses Association: Emergency Nursing Care Curriculum, 4th ed. Philadelphia, WB Saunders, 1994.

Kelly W: Rapid Assessment. Springhouse, PA, Springhouse Corporation, 1991.

Kitt S, Selfridge-Thomas J, Pruehl J, Kaiser J: Emergency Nursing: A Physiologic and Clinical Perspective, 2nd ed. Philadelphia, WB Saunders, 1995.

Chapter 2
Cardiovascular Emergencies

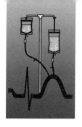

LEAD PLACEMENT

- Monitor leads are often colored to facilitate appropriate placement.
- For the purposes of this chapter, the following "colors" will be used:
  - White = Negative ($-$)
  - Red = Positive ($+$)
  - Black = Ground (g)

Lead I

- Red ($+$) = below left clavicle
- White ($-$) = below right clavicle
- Black (g) = lowest palpable rib, left midclavicular line

Lead II (Common for Monitoring)

- Red ($+$) = lowest palpable rib, left midclavicular line
- White ($-$) = below right clavicle
- Black (g) = below left clavicle

Lead III

- Red ($+$) = lowest palpable rib, left midclavicular line

- White ($-$) = below left clavicle
- Black (g) = right side of chest, lowest palpable rib

MCL₁ (Modified Chest Lead That Simulates V₁)

- Red ($+$) = fourth intercostal space, right sternal border
- White ($-$) = below left clavicle
- Black (g) = below right clavicle

MCL₆ (Modified Chest Lead That Simulates V₆)

- Red ($+$) = fifth intercostal space, left midaxillary line
- White ($-$) = below left clavicle
- Black (g) = below right clavicle

12-LEAD EKG

- Precordial lead placement is summarized in Table 2–1.
- Limb leads are I, II, and III, and the three augmented leads are aV_R, aV_L, and aV_F. These leads are placed on the patient's arms and legs with the ground lead placed on the patient's right leg.

RIGHT-SIDED 12-LEAD EKG

- Indications
  - Suspected acute right ventricular infarction
  - Almost always in the presence of acute inferior or posterior myocardial infarction
  - In rare instances manifested by ST depression only in V_1–V_3

Table 2–1. Precordial Lead Placement for 12-Lead EKG

Lead	Electrode Placement
V_1	Fourth intercostal space at the right border of the sternum
V_2	Fourth intercostal space at the left border of the sternum
V_3	Midway between locations V_2 and V_4
V_4	At the midclavicular line in the fifth intercostal space
V_5	At the anterior axillary line on the same horizontal level as V_4
V_6	At the midaxillary line on the same horizontal level as V_4 and V_5

- Lead placement is the mirror image of a standard 12-lead EKG.
  - Precordial lead placement is summarized in Table 2–2.
  - Limb leads are I, II, and III, and the three augmented leads are aV_R, aV_L, and aV_F. These leads are placed on the patient's arms and legs with the ground lead placed on the patient's right leg.

CARDIAC TAMPONADE

- Pericardial sac fills with blood.
- Intrapericardial pressure increases.
- Ventricular venous filling decreases.
- Cardiac output (CO) decreases.
- Cardiac tamponade is due to blunt or penetrating trauma.

Table 2–2. Precordial Lead Placement for Right-Sided 12-Lead EKG

Lead	Electrode Placement
RV_1	Fourth intercostal space at the left border of the sternum
RV_2	Fourth intercostal space at the right border of the sternum
RV_3	Midway between locations RV_2 and RV_4
RV_4	At the midclavicular line in the fifth intercostal space
RV_5	At the anterior axillary line on the same horizontal level as RV_4
RV_6	At the midaxillary line on the same horizontal level as RV_4 and RV_5

- If not treated immediately, tamponade can lead to cardiac arrest.

Signs and Symptoms of Cardiac Tamponade

- Beck's triad
  - Hypotension
  - Muffled heart tones
  - Tachycardia
- Neck vein distention
- Pulsus paradoxus: a fall in systolic blood pressure during inspiration >3–10 mm Hg

Procedures for Treatment
(see Chapter 18)

ISCHEMIA

- Inverted T wave
- May also have ST segment depression

- Due to a temporary interruption of myocardial blood flow

INJURY

- ST segment elevation
- Signifies an acute process
- Due to prolonged interruption of myocardial blood flow
- Greater than 0.1 mV (one small square on the vertical axis) may be significant for injury

INFARCTION (see Table 2–3)

- Q waves may be pathologic.
- Small Q waves may be normal in V_5, V_6, I, and aV_L.
- Abnormal Q wave must be 0.04 second (one small square on the horizontal axis).
- Abnormal Q wave depth is greater than ⅓ of the QRS height in lead III.

Table 2–3. Sites of Infarction

Wall	Leads	Artery
Inferior	II, III, aV_F	Right coronary (RCA)
Lateral	I, aV_L, V_5, V_6	Circumflex, branch of left anterior descending (LAD)
Anterior	V_1, V_2, V_3, V_4	Left coronary
Posterior	V_1, V_2, V_3	RCA, circumflex
Apical	V_3, V_4, V_5, V_6	LAD, RCA
Anterolateral	I, aV_L, V_4, V_5, V_6	LAD, circumflex
Anteroseptal	V_1, V_2, V_3	LAD

ASSESSMENT OF CHEST PAIN

- PQRST mnemonic is easy to remember. PQRST is also normal component of an EKG waveform.
  - P = Provokes
  - Q = Quality of pain
  - R = Region and/or Radiation
  - S = Severity
  - T = Timing
- The severity of chest pain can be assessed by using
  - 1–10 pain scale (1 = minimal pain, 10 = worst pain ever suffered)
  - Wong-Baker Faces of Pain Rating Scale for those with language or speech barriers (see Fig. 2–1)

CAUSES OF CHEST PAIN

- Heart
  - Angina
  - Acute myocardial infarction
  - Pericarditis
  - Cardiac tamponade (traumatic or postoperative)
  - Dissecting aortic aneurysm
- Lung
  - Chest wall pain

Figure 2–1. The Wong-Baker Faces of Pain Rating Scale. (From Wong DL: Whaley & Wong's Nursing Care of Infants and Children, 5th ed. St. Louis, Mosby-Year Book, 1995.)

- Costochondritis
- Pleurisy
- Pulmonary embolus
- Spontaneous pneumothorax
- Traumatic pneumothorax and/or hemothorax
- Abdomen
  - Esophageal reflux or spasm
  - Hiatal hernia
  - Peptic ulcer disease
  - Cholecystitis
  - Pancreatitis
- Psychologic problems: acute anxiety

EDEMA

- Excess accumulation of fluid in the interstitial spaces
- Two types of edema
  - Pitting (leaves indentation upon pressure)
    - 0–¼ inch = mild (1+) (+)
    - ¼–½ inch = moderate (2+) (++)
    - ½–1 inch or more = severe (3+) (+++)
  - Nonpitting
- Important to assess the extent of edema. For example:
  - Foot
  - Foot to ankle
  - Ankle to knee
  - Foot to thigh
  - Sacrum

ADVANCED CARDIAC LIFE SUPPORT TREATMENT

- All treatment guidelines are from the American Medical Association.[1]

Universal Algorithm for Adult Emergency Cardiac Care (ECC)

- Assess responsiveness.
- If the patient is unresponsive, activate the EMS system.
- Call for defibrillator.
- Assess breathing (open airway, look, listen, and feel).
- If the patient is not breathing, give two slow breaths.
- Assess circulation: if no pulse, start CPR.

Ventricular Fibrillation/Pulseless Ventricular Tachycardia

- Check ABCs.
- Perform CPR until defibrillator attached.
- Confirm ventricular fibrillation (VF) or ventricular tachycardia (VT) present on defibrillator/monitor; confirm no pulse.
- Defibrillate up to three times, if needed, for persistent VF/VT (200 J, 200–300 J, 360 J).
- If the rhythm after the first three shocks is persistent, or if there's recurrent VF/VT, continue CPR.
- Intubate at once.
- Obtain IV access.
- Administer epinephrine 1 mg IV push; repeat every 3 to 5 minutes.
- Defibrillate at 360 J within 30–60 seconds.
- Administer medications of probable benefit in persistent or recurrent VF (lidocaine, bretylium, magnesium sulfate, procainamide, or sodium bicarbonate).

- Defibrillate at 360 J within 30–60 seconds after each dose of medication.
- Pattern should be "drug-shock, drug-shock."

Ventricular Tachycardia: Clinically Stable

- Check ABCs.
- Obtain venous access.
- Administer lidocaine initial dose of 1–1.5 mg/kg IV push.
- Administer lidocaine 0.5–0.75 mg/kg 5–10 minutes later.
- Lidocaine total loading dose is 3 mg/kg.
- A lidocaine drip of 2–4 mg/minute should be continued if arrhythmia is converted.
- Procainamide 20–30 mg/minute until:
  - 17 mg/kg has been given
  - Hypotension
  - More than 50% widening of the QRS complex
  - Suppression of the arrhythmia
- Administer procainamide infusion at 1–4 mg/minute if the arrhythmia is converted.
- Administer bretylium 5–10 mg/kg over 8–10 minutes.
- If bretylium converts the arrhythmia, complete the loading dose and start a continuous infusion at a rate of 1–2 mg/minute.

Ventricular Tachycardia: Hemodynamically Unstable

- Check ABCs.
- Obtain venous access.
- Unstable tachycardia = hypotension, shortness of

breath, chest pain, altered consciousness, or
pulmonary edema.
- Prepare for immediate cardioversion if ventricular
rate is more than 150 beats/minute.
  - May give brief trial of medications based on
    specific arrhythmias
  - Immediate cardioversion generally not needed
    for rates less than 150 beats/minute
- Premedicate whenever possible.
- Synchronize cardioversion (treat polymorphic VT
  like VF: 200 J, 200–300 J, 360 J).

Symptomatic Bradycardia

- Check ABCs.
- Obtain venous access.
- Administer atropine 0.5 to 1.0 mg IV push and in
  repeat doses in 3 to 5 minutes up to a total of
  0.04 mg/kg.
- Place transcutaneous pacemaker if available.
- Administer dopamine, 5–20 µg/kg per minute, IV
  infusion.
- Administer epinephrine, 2–10 µg/kg per minute,
  IV infusion.
- Administer isoproterenol (if at all) with extreme
  caution, IV infusion.

Atrial Fibrillation/Atrial Flutter

- Check ABCs.
- Obtain venous access.
- Consider use of
  - Diltiazem
  - Beta-blockers
  - Verapamil
  - Digoxin
  - Procainamide

- Quinidine
- Anticoagulants
- Synchronize cardioversion if patient becomes unstable or fails to convert.

Paroxysmal Supraventricular Tachycardia (PSVT)

- Check ABCs.
- Obtain venous access.
- Perform vagal maneuvers.
- Administer adenosine 6 mg rapid IV push over 1–3 seconds.
- Administer adenosine 12 mg rapid IV push over 1–3 seconds (may repeat once in 1–2 minutes).
- Narrow complex width with normal blood pressure, administer
  - Verapamil 2.5–5 mg IV (repeat in 15–30 minutes)
  - Consider digoxin, beta-blockers, diltiazem
- For wide complex with normal blood pressure, administer
  - Lidocaine 1–1.5 mg/kg IV push
  - Procainamide 20–30 mg/minute (total 17 mg/kg)
- Synchronize cardioversion if low blood pressure or patient becomes unstable.

Asystole

- Check ABCs.
- Perform CPR.
- Intubate at once.
- Obtain IV access.
- Confirm asystole in more than one lead.
- Consider possible causes:

- Hypoxia
- Hyperkalemia
- Hypokalemia
- Preexisting acidosis
- Drug overdose
- Hypothermia
- Consider immediate transcutaneous pacing
- Epinephrine 1 mg IV push, repeat every 3–5 minutes. If this fails, can use
  - *intermediate* dosing: 2–5 mg IV push every 3–5 minutes
  - *escalating* dosing: 1 mg–3 mg–5 mg IV push 3 minutes apart, *or*
  - *high* dosing: 0.1 mg/kg IV push every 3–5 minutes
- Atropine 1 mg IV, repeat every 3–5 min up to a total of 0.04 mg/kg
- Consider termination of efforts

Pulseless Electrical Activity (PEA)

- Identify PEA and treat the possible causes.
- A helpful mnemonic is **PEA PATCHHHH**, which covers most causes of PEA.
  - P = Pulmonary embolism
  - A = Acidosis
  - T = Tension pneumothorax
  - C = Cardiac tamponade
  - H = Hypovolemia
  - H = Hypoxia
  - H = Hypothermia
  - H = Hyperkalemia
- Check ABCs.
- Obtain venous access.
- Perform CPR.

- Consider the causes:
  - Hypovolemia (give a volume infusion)
  - Hypoxia (ventilate)
  - Hypothermia
  - Hyperkalemia
  - Cardiac tamponade (pericardiocentesis)
  - Tension pneumothorax (needle decompression)
  - Massive pulmonary embolism (surgery, thrombolytics)
  - Drug overdose
  - Acidosis
  - Massive acute myocardial infarction

Reference

1. American Medical Association: Guidelines for cardiopul-monary resuscitation and emergency cardiac care. JAMA. 268:2199–2241, 1992

Chapter 3

Communicable/ Infectious Diseases

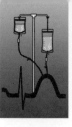

COMMUNICABLE DISEASES

- Important factors in diagnosing and treating communicable diseases include incubation period as well as mode of transmission (see Table 3–1).

HIV-RELATED INFECTIONS SEEN IN THE ED

Candidiasis

- Fungal infection
- Most common in oral cavity and esophagus; may also see skin, rectal, and vaginal lesions
- Treatment may include clotrimazole, nystatin, ketoconazole, fluconazole, itraconazole

Coccidioidomycosis*

- Fungal disease
- Endemic in Southwest United States, Northern Mexico, parts of Central and South America (check travel to these areas)

---

*Reportable diseases for AIDS cases.

- Six clinical categories, symptoms depend on organ system involved:
  - Focal pulmonary
  - Diffuse pulmonary
  - Skin
  - Meningitis
  - Lymph node or liver
  - Positive serology
- Definitive treatment is unknown; treatment may include amphotericin B, fluconazole, itraconazole

*Cryptococcus neoformans**

- Fungal infection
- May cause pulmonary, central nervous system, or disseminated infection (most common is meningitis)
- Diagnosis: serum and cerebrospinal fluid cryptococcal antigen test is very sensitive
- Treatment: amphotericin B with or without flucytosine (5FU); fluconazole

Cryptosporidium, Isospora belli,* Microsporida

- Protozoan infections responsible for diarrhea and abdominal pain
- Treatment includes symptomatic relief by use of antidiarrheal drugs and fluids; may also use paromomycin, azithromycin, octreotide, TMP/SMX, pyrimethamine and folinic acid, metronidazole, and albendazole

---

*Reportable diseases for AIDS cases.

Cytomegalovirus (CMV)*

- Virus (a member of the beta herpes virus subfamily)
- May cause
  - Chorioretinitis (unilateral visual field loss, blurring of vision, scotomata)
  - Gastrointestinal disease (abdominal pain, diarrhea)
  - Pneumonia (interstitial infiltrates on chest x-ray, hypoxia)
  - Less frequently seen: central nervous system and adrenal disease
- Treatment may include ganciclovir (DHPG), foscarnet sodium

Herpes Simplex (HSV)*

- Virus
- Common sites: genital, rectal, orolabial, and esophageal
- Signs and symptoms: pain, ulcerations
- Treatment may include acyclovir, foscarnet sodium, topical silver sulfadiazine

Histoplasmosis*

- Fungal infection
- Endemic to South Central United States, South America (check recent travel)
- Signs and symptoms reflect diffuse infection: fever, weight loss, skin lesions, adenopathy, respiratory complaints, hepatosplenomegaly
- Treatment: amphotericin

---

*Reportable diseases for AIDS cases.

Kaposi's Sarcoma*

- Malignancy (epidemiologic evidence points towards an infectious agent)
- Symptoms: lesions, painless nodules or macules, pigmented red, purple, or brown in skin or oral cavity (early), then involvement in GI tract, lungs, lymphatics, and genital area
- Treatment: Chemotherapeutic agents are the standard approach.

*Mycobacterium tuberculosis (MTB)**

- Bacterial infection
- All persons with HIV infection should receive yearly tuberculin skin testing
- Among cases of multiple drug-resistant MTB (MDRTB), most occur in HIV-infected persons.
- Tuberculosis (TB) infection present: positive purified protein derivative (PPD), may have negative cultures, negative chest x-ray
- Active disease present: positive cultures, *or* positive PPD and positive chest x-ray
- Signs and symptoms are nonspecific: fever, nightsweats, weight loss, cough, hemoptysis
- May be pulmonary or extrapulmonary, and findings vary with the organ system involved
- PPD: 5 mm of induration or more is considered positive in HIV-infected persons
- Treatment: positive PPD *or* history of positive PPD, isoniazid (INH), and pyridoxine
- Active MTB: INH with pyridoxine, rifampin, pyrazinamide, and ethambutol *or* streptomycin for

---

*Reportable diseases for AIDS cases.

23

8 weeks. Follow with INH and rifampin. (Other options are available.)

*Pneumocystis carinii**

- Protozoan or possibly a fungal infection of lungs
- Signs and symptoms: fever, inflammation, impaired gas exchange, fatigue, weight loss, diarrhea, cough, shortness of breath, dyspnea on exertion
- Diagnosis: CD4 (T-4 lymphocyte) counts usually less than 200, bilateral interstitial infiltrates on chest x-ray, increased alveolar-arterial gradient (>35 mm Hg) and hypoxia (Po_2 <80 mm Hg) on arterial blood gases
- Treatment may include the following medications: TMP/SMX, dapsone, atovaquone, clindamycin
- Oxygen, monitoring, and corticosteroids for severe disease

Progressive Multifocal Leukoencephalopathy (PML)*

- Caused by the JC virus
- Selective demyelination of white matter of the brain
- Signs and symptoms: slowly progressive neurologic dysfunction (dementia, visual deficits, abnormal gait, hemiparesis, ataxia, sensory deficits, difficulty with speech and language)
- Diagnosis: focal or diffuse lesions on computed tomography (CT) scan (magnetic resonance imaging [MRI] may be more sensitive); lumbar puncture (LP) usually shows normal cerebrospinal

*Reportable diseases for AIDS cases.

fluid (CSF) (LP may be helpful in excluding other conditions)
- Treatment: no proven therapy; cytosine arabinoside may be effective

*Toxoplasma gondii**

- Protozoan infection
- Cats and other animals serve as reservoir for the organism
- Signs and symptoms: most common site is intracranial (headaches, confusion, fever, seizures, poor coordination, abnormal gait; focal neurologic changes are most common physical findings)
- Diagnosis: ring-enhancing lesions are most evident on CT after double-dose delayed contrast study (MRI may be more sensitive); LP performed after CT (to prevent potential herniation) may be normal.
- Treatment may include sulfadiazine, clindamycin, pyrimethamine, folinic acid

---

*Reportable diseases for AIDS cases.

Table 3–1. Selected Communicable Diseases Seen in Emergency Departments

Disease	Incubation Period	Description, Transmission (T), and Duration (D)
AIDS	Unknown	See CDC Guidelines for reportable AIDS cases for HIV infected persons; T: sexual contact, blood/body fluids
Candidiasis	2–5 days	Communicable for duration of lesions
Cat scratch fever	3–14 days from inoculation to lesions	T: through scratch, bite, lick, or other exposure to healthy cat; no direct transmission from person to person
Chickenpox	14–21 days	D: 5–20 days; contagious from 1 day before eruption until 6–7 days after lesions are crusted; rash begins as small, red macules, progresses to papules, and then to vesicles
Chlamydia	5–10 days or more	T: sexual contact

Conjunctivitis	24–72 hours	T: direct or indirect contact with discharge from the infected eye
Cytomegalovirus (CMV)	3–8 weeks after blood transfusion 3–12 weeks after delivery (neonatal)	Virus excreted in urine or saliva
Diarrhea (see gastroenteritis)		
Diphtheria	2–5 days	Characteristic lesion is patches of adherent grayish membrane with surrounding inflammation; usually in oropharynx; primarily found in unimmunized persons and communicable for average of 2 weeks
Erythema infectiosum (fifth disease)	6–14 days	Macular rash gives "slapped cheeks" appearance; lacy rash on arms and legs; may recur if exposed to strong sunlight

Table continued on following page

27

Table 3–1. Selected Communicable Diseases Seen in Emergency Departments (Continued)

Disease	Incubation Period	Description, Transmission (T), and Duration (D)
Food poisoning Staphylococcal	30 min to 7 hrs	Frequently found in pastries, custards, salad dressings, sandwiches, sliced meats that have remained at room temperature for several hours
Botulism	12–36 hours	Characterized by CNS manifestations such as ptosis, visual difficulty, followed by descending symmetrical flaccid paralysis; vomiting and diarrhea may be present initially; frequently found in improperly canned foods
Clostridium	6–24 hours	Sudden onset of colic followed by diarrhea; frequently found in food contaminated by soil or feces; associated with inadequately heated meats

Gastroenteritis (*diarrhea due to E. coli*)	12–72 hours	Perfuse watery diarrhea, abdominal cramping, vomiting; T: contaminated feces; D: symptoms usually last <3–5 days
Campylobacter	1–10 days	Diarrhea, abdominal pain, fever, nausea, vomiting; T: organism found in food, unpasteurized milk; usually self-limited within 1–4 days. If not treated with antibiotics, organism is excreted for 2–7 weeks
Rotaviral enteritis	48 hours	Seen in infants and young children; characterized by diarrhea and vomiting; T: fecal-oral or fecal-respiratory
Viral	24–48 hours	Self-limited, mild disease; nausea, vomiting, diarrhea, abdominal pain, myalgia, low-grade fever; T: unknown, probably fecal-oral route

Table continued on following page

Table 3-1. Selected Communicable Diseases Seen in Emergency Departments (Continued)

Disease	Incubation Period	Description, Transmission (T), and Duration (D)
Giardiasis	5–25 days	Protozoan disease; diarrhea, steatorrhea, abdominal cramps, fatigue, weight loss; T: ingestion of cysts in fecally contaminated water or food
Salmonella	6–72 hours	Symptoms include headache, abdominal pain, nausea, vomiting, and diarrhea; T: by ingestion of infected food or feces-contaminated foods including raw eggs, raw milk, meat, and poultry; also pet turtles and chicks
Gonococcal	2–7 days	T: sexual contact; D: communicable for months if untreated

Hepatitis		
A (infectious hepatitis)	15–50 days	T: fecal-oral, person to person
B (serum hepatitis)	45–180 days	Blood, saliva, semen and vaginal fluids may be infectious; T: percutaneous or permucosal exposure
C (post-transfusion non-A, non-B)	15–160 days	T: contaminated blood products, parenteral route
D (delta virus)	15–64 days	T: percutaneous exposures; infection only in presence of hepatitis B infection
E (enteric non-A, non-B)	14–63 days	T: fecal-oral route; frequently associated with poor sanitation
Herpes	2–12 days	Characterized by localized primary lesion, latency, and a tendency to localized recurrence; T: direct contact
Impetigo	N/A	Bacterial (*Staphylococcus* or *Streptococcus*) infection; vesicular lesions; advances to yellow crust on a red base
Influenza	24–72 hours	Viral; T: direct contact with droplet infection; virus may persist for hours in dried mucus

Table continued on following page

31

Table 3-1. Selected Communicable Diseases Seen in Emergency Departments *(Continued)*

Disease	Incubation Period	Description, Transmission (T), and Duration (D)
Kawasaki syndrome	Unknown	Unknown cause; D: 6–8 weeks; red maculopapular lesions; progresses to pruritic wheals; desquamation occurs within 2–7 days
Legionnaires' disease	2–10 days	Bacterial disease characterized by anorexia, myalgia, headache, fever, chills, cough, abdominal pain and diarrhea; T: airborne
Lice (pediculosis)	Eggs hatch in 7 days	Infestation of hairy parts of body; T: direct contact with an infested person
Lyme disease	3–32 days after tick exposure	A tick-borne spirochetal disease with distinctive skin lesions; lesions may be accompanied by malaise, fatigue, fever, headache, stiff neck, arthralgias, or lymphadenopathy; check recent possible tick exposure

Measles		
Rubeola (hard measles, red measles)	10–20 days	Contagious from 4 days before to 5 days after rash appears; D: 10–15 days; rash is reddish macules; begins on face and spreads downward; within 1–2 days rash is confluent
Rubella, (German measles)	14–21 days	Contagious from 7 days before to 5 days after rash appears; D: 3–4 days; fever uncommon; rash is macular pink to red, begins on head and spreads downward
Meningitis		
Viral	Variable	Characterized by sudden onset of febrile illness with signs and symptoms of meningeal involvement; CSF shows increased protein, normal sugar, no bacteria

Table continued on following page

33

Table 3–1. Selected Communicable Diseases Seen in Emergency Departments (Continued)

Disease	Incubation Period	Description, Transmission (T), and Duration (D)
Bacterial	2–10 days	70% of cases occur in children <5 years old. Includes both meningococcal and *Haemophilus* meningitis; T: direct contact including droplets and discharges from nose and throat
Mononucleosis	4–6 weeks	Infectious agent is Epstein-Barr virus; T: person to person by oropharyngeal route; fever, sore throat, lymphadenopathy are characteristic
Mumps	2–3 weeks	Infective up to 7 days before and 9 days after parotitis; viral disease characterized by fever, swelling, and tenderness of 1 or more salivary glands

Pertussis (whooping cough)	7–10 days	Paroxysms characterized by repeated violent coughs followed by high-pitched inspiratory "whoop"; T: direct contact with respiratory discharges of infected persons
Rabies	2–8 weeks	T: virus-laden saliva of a rabid animal; D: 2–6 days; death (if not treated) is due to respiratory paralysis
Rocky mountain spotted fever	3–14 days	Characterized by sudden onset of fever, malaise, deep muscle pain, headache, chills, and conjunctival infection; rash appears approximately the third day; T: bite of an infected tick

Table continued on following page

Table 3-1. Selected Communicable Diseases Seen in Emergency Departments (Continued)

Disease	Incubation Period	Description, Transmission (T), and Duration (D)
Scabies	2–6 weeks	T: direct skin-to-skin contact by mite infestation; the mite penetration is visible as papules or vesicles, or as tiny linear burrows containing mites and their eggs
Scarlet fever	1–7 days	Contagious during incubation period; Bacterial Group A streptococcal infection; fine raised maculopapular rash; red strawberry tongue
Streptococcal disease	1–3 days	Frequent cause of sore throat due to Group A β-hemolytic bacteria; T: direct or intimate contact with infected person

Disease	Incubation period	Description
Syphilis	10 days to 10 weeks	Characterized by primary lesion (chancroid), a secondary eruption involving skin and mucous membranes and periods of latency if untreated; T: sexual contact
Tetanus (lockjaw)	3–21 days	T: tetanus spores introduced into the body by a puncture wound contaminated with soil or feces
Trichomoniasis	4–20 days	Genitourinary disease characterized by punctate lesions and a perfuse, thin, foamy yellowish discharge with foul odor; T: sexual contact; motile parasite infection
Tuberculosis	4–12 weeks	T: exposure to the bacilli in airborne droplets from sputum of infected persons; communicable as long as the bacilli are being discharged in the sputum

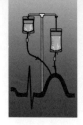

Chapter 4

ENT Emergencies

PROBLEMS OF THE EAR

Otitis Media

- Tympanic membrane (TM) may be bulging, red, or pink (normal TM is shiny, pearly gray, and translucent)
- Common in infants and children, may also be seen in adults

CAUSES OF OTITIS MEDIA

- Bacteria enter the middle ear
- Forceful nose-blowing forcing exudate into the middle ear
- Effusion
- Otitic barotrauma (e.g., aircraft landings)
- Trauma to the TM (e.g., rupture of the TM)

COMPLICATIONS OF UNTREATED OTITIS MEDIA

- Hearing loss
- Abscess (neck or intracranial)
- Mastoiditis
- Meningitis

- Antibiotics
- Analgesics
- Thorough discharge instructions

External Otitis

- Inflammation of the external ear
- Sometimes called *swimmer's ear*

- Gram-negative organisms
- Fungi
- Dermatosis

- Anti-inflammatory otic solutions
- Use of an ear wick often necessary to instill medications into the swollen ear canal
- Instructions regarding no swimming or immersion of ear

Ruptured Tympanic Membrane

- Can result from chronic infections or trauma
- A tear or perforation of the TM is visible via otoscope

- History of trauma or recent infection
- Discharge from ear canal

- Decreased hearing
- Fever

- Oral analgesics
- Referral for follow-up

Foreign Body in the Ear

- Small objects such as rocks, beads, vegetable matter
- Insects crawling or flying into the ear canal (cockroaches, mosquitoes, beetles, flies, etc.)
- Can see object or insect with an otoscope

*EMERGENCY INTERVENTIONS
INCLUDE*

- Instillation of 2% xylocaine solution into canal containing a live insect may stun or kill it.
- Irrigate the ear with warm tap water or saline (body temperature). Never use cold water as an irrigant for foreign body removal (may stimulate vomiting).
- For irrigation use a standard ear syringe, commercial irrigation set, or a 20–30 cc syringe with an IV angiocath (shortened and the stylet removed).

NASAL CONDITIONS SEEN IN THE ED

Epistaxis

- Most common type is the anterior epistaxis

CAUSES OF ANTERIOR EPISTAXIS

- Trauma
- Foreign bodies

- Nose picking
- Dry nasal passages

CAUSES OF POSTERIOR EPISTAXIS

- Hypertension
- Atherosclerosis of vessels
- Age (more common in the elderly)

EMERGENCY INTERVENTIONS FOR EPISTAXIS ABATEMENT

- Topical vasoconstrictors
- Cautery
  - Silver nitrate
  - Electric
  - Battery-operated, single patient use (disposable) cauterizer
- Packing
  - Petrolatum gauze
  - Hemostatic material (gelfoam)
  - Nasal balloon catheters

Nasal Fractures

- Greenstick
- Linear
- Comminuted
- Causes include
  - Blunt trauma, most common
  - Epistaxis common due to Kiesselbach's triangle
    - A thin, highly vascular area of the nasal septum that receives its blood supply from the internal and external carotid artery system
    - May be the site of perforation and epistaxis

Nasal Septal Hematoma

- An emergent condition
- If untreated can lead to
  - Airway obstruction
  - Septal necrosis
  - Permanent deformity of the nose
- ENT consult usually necessary for evacuation and treatment of the hematoma

Nasal Foreign Bodies

- Small objects (rocks, beads, vegetable matter)
- Usually painless
- Organic matter may break down or germinate
- Odor is common
- Can see with an otoscope and use of a nasal speculum
- Commonly removed with forceps (e.g., bayonet) or suction

CONDITIONS OF THE THROAT

- Pharyngitis
- Inflammation of the musculomembranous tube situated at the back of the nose, mouth, and larynx

Frequent Causes of Throat Conditions

- Beta-hemolytic streptococcus
- Staphylococci
- Pneumococci
- *Haemophilus influenzae*
- May also be viral or fungal

Emergency Interventions for Throat Conditions

- Antibiotics as indicated
- Antipyretics
- Local analgesics
- Salt-water gargles

Laryngitis

- Inflammation of the mucous membranes of the larynx
- May be
  - Acute
  - Chronic
  - Catarrhal
  - Suppurative
  - Croupous
  - Tuberculous
  - Syphilitic
- Emergency interventions include
  - Antibiotics as indicated
  - Local analgesics
  - Voice rest

Tonsillitis

- Inflammation of the tonsils
- Usually caused by
  - Streptococci
  - Other bacteria
  - Viruses
  - Fungi
- May be
  - Acute
  - Chronic
  - Recurring

- Tonsils can become cryptic (with concealed pockets)
- Can have foreign bodies embedded in the crypts:
  - Fingernails
  - Seeds
  - Fishbones
- Emergency interventions include
  - Antibiotics
  - Antipyretics
  - Local analgesics

Tonsillar Abscess

- An abscess forming in acute tonsillitis around one or both tonsils
- Also known as "quinsy"
- Characterized by
  - Enlarged tonsil(s)
  - Edema
  - Dysphagia or drooling
  - Muffled voice due to edema
  - Pus on tonsil(s)
- Emergency interventions
  - Continous assessment of airway patency
  - Emergency airway equipment readily available
  - Parenteral antibiotics
  - IV hydration
  - Analgesics
  - Antipyretics
  - Aspiration of abscess

Epiglottitis

- Inflammation of the epiglottis
- Less common, but a true emergency
- Seen primarily in pediatric patients

SIGNS AND SYMPTOMS OF EPIGLOTTITIS

- Dyspnea
- Inspiratory stridor
- Use of accessory muscles
- Fever
- Drooling
- Tachycardia
- Dysphagia
- Muffled voice
- Sore throat
- Possible hypoxemia when the swollen epiglottis obstructs the airway

CAUSE OF EPIGLOTTITIS

- *Haemophilus influenzae* type B pneumococci
- Group A streptococci

EMERGENCY INTERVENTIONS FOR EPIGLOTTITIS

- Maintain a child in an upright position (child may remain in caregiver's lap).
- Avoid agitating patient.
- Do not insert anything into the mouth (tongue blade, oral thermometer).
- Do not attempt to visualize the pharynx.
- Have intubation or cricothyroidotomy tray at bedside.

Bibliography

Bates B: A Guide to Physical Examination, 3rd ed. Philadelphia, JB Lippincott, 1983.

Emergency Nurses Association: Emergency Nursing Core Curriculum, 4th ed. Philadelphia, WB Saunders, 1994.

Thompson J, Bowers A: Clinical Manual of Health Assessment. St. Louis, CV Mosby, 1980.

Chapter 5
Endocrine Emergencies

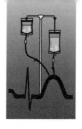

CONDITIONS RELATED TO DIABETES MELLITUS

- Type I (insulin dependent, see Table 5–1)
- Type II (noninsulin dependent)

Diabetic Ketoacidosis (DKA)

- Caused by insulin deficit
- Produces hyperglycemia, lipolysis, and protein catabolism
- Glucose is prevented from entering into the cells and accumulates in the serum

MANIFESTATIONS OF DIABETIC KETOACIDOSIS

- Produces osmotic diuresis
- Results in systemic dehydration
- Lipolysis and protein catabolism produce cellular energy. Ketones are the byproduct.
- Hyperventilation occurs to compensate for metabolic acidosis.

TREATMENT FOR DIABETIC KETOACIDOSIS

- Initial IV infusion of regular insulin (20–50 units)
- Followed by single subcutaneous injections, IV injections, or IV infusions of insulin

Table 5-1. Types of Insulin

Name	Onset	Peak	Duration
Regular (Humulin-R, Novolin R, Iletin I, Velosulin)	0.5–1 hr	2–5 hrs	5–8 hrs
Prompt insulin zinc suspension (Semilente Insulin, Semilente Iletin I, Semilente purified pork)	1–2 hrs	5–10 hrs	12–16 hrs
Isophane insulin suspension (NPH, Humulin-N, Insulatard NPH, Insulatard NPH Human)	1–2 hrs	4–12 hrs	24–48 hrs
Insulin zinc suspension (Humulin-L, Lente Insulin, Lente Iletin I and II, Novolin L)	1–3 hrs	6–15 hrs	24–28 hrs
Protamine zinc insulin (PZI) suspension (Protamine Zinc Iletin I and II)	4–8 hrs	14–24 hrs	36 hrs or more
Extended insulin zinc suspension (Ultralente)	4–8 hrs	10–30 hrs	36 hrs or more
Isophane insulin suspension (Mixtard Novolin 70/30)	0.25–1 hr	2–8 hrs	24 hrs

- Typical goal is to deliver 5–10 units of insulin/hour depending on the response to the initial dose
- For insulin infusions: Prime the IV tubing and discard the first 50 mL of solution (insulin binds to plastic IV tubing).
- IV therapy
  - 0.9% NaCl rapidly for fluid volume depletion
  - $D_5.45\%$ after hypovolemia and hyperglycemia are treated
- Sodium bicarbonate if pH is less than 7.1
- Potassium added to the IV fluids if hypokalemia is present

Hyperglycemic Hyperosmolar Nonketotic Coma (HHNC)

- Occurs in Type II diabetics
- Patient may have history of impaired renal, cardiac, or cerebral function

MANIFESTATIONS OF HHNC

- Dehydration due to hyperglycemia
- Osmotic diuresis occurs as in DKA
- No ketoacidosis due to presence of enough endogenous insulin
- Infection, sepsis, or stroke is often present.
- Serum glucose levels are very high (often >1000 mg/dL).

TREATMENT FOR HHNC

- IV fluid volume replacement
- Potassium added to IV fluids for hypokalemia
- Insulin may or may not be necessary

Hypoglycemia

- Caused by an oversupply of insulin
- Underproduction of glucose

MANIFESTATIONS OF HYPOGLYCEMIA

- Glucose less than 35 mg/dL results in hypoxia
- Coma due to the lack of oxygen extraction by the brain

TREATMENT FOR HYPOGLYCEMIA

- Oral glucose administration for less severe cases, but patient must be awake and able to swallow
- Dextrose IV push
  - Adults: dextrose 50%
  - Children: dextrose 25%
  - Neonates: dextrose 10%
  - IV fluids
  - If the patient has an insulin pump, it must be turned off.

THYROID CONDITIONS

Thyroid Storm

- Hypermetabolic crisis
- Overactive thyroid gland
- Overproduction of thyroid hormones

MANIFESTATIONS OF THYROID STORM

- Elevated temperature greater than 37°C (may be as high as 41°C)
- Rapid tachycardia (may be as high as 200–300 beats/min)

- CNS symptoms
  - Tremors
  - Restlessness
  - Agitation
  - Labile mood
  - Manic/psychotic behavior
- Cardiovascular symptoms
  - Increased stroke volume
  - Increased systolic blood pressure
  - Increased cardiac output
  - Arrhythmias
  - CHF
- GI dysfunction
  - Diarrhea
  - Nausea and vomiting
  - Abdominal cramps
  - Jaundice

TREATMENT FOR THYROID STORM

- ABCs
- Fluid resuscitation
- Reduction in thyroid hormone levels
  - Lugol's solution (iodine)
  - Sodium iodide, slow IV infusion via pump
  - Beta-blockers to counteract thyroid hormone effects
  - Antipyretics for fever control

Myxedema Coma

- Rare complication of hypothyroidism
- Results in encephalopathy and respiratory depression

FACTORS PRECIPITATING MYXEDEMA COMA

- Upper respiratory infection (URI)
- Other infection

- Trauma
- Stress
- Surgery
- Anesthesia
- CHF
- CVA
- GI bleed

*SIGNS/SYMPTOMS OF MYXEDEMA
COMA: "HYPO" SIGNS*

- Hyporesponsiveness
- Hypoventilation
- Hypotension
- Hypo(brady)cardia
- Hypothermia
- Hypotonia
- Hyponatremia
- Hypoglycemia
- Hypoadrenalism

TREATMENT FOR MYXEDEMA COMA

- ABCs
- IV fluids
- Thyroxine 100–500 μg IV slowly or
  triiodothyronine

ADRENAL CRISIS (ADDISONIAN CRISIS)

- Caused by the destruction of adrenal cortex
- Cortisol and aldosterone are inadequate
- Causes of adrenal cortex destruction or crisis
  include
  - Tumor
  - Infiltration

- TB infection
- Hemorrhage
- Bilateral adrenalectomies
- Drugs
- Iatrogenic insufficiency
- Signs and symptoms of adrenal crisis include
  - Hypotension
  - Hypovolemia
  - Hyponatremia
  - Hyperkalemia
  - Shock
  - Fever
  - Abdominal pain
  - Nausea, vomiting, diarrhea
  - Weakness
  - EKG abnormalities
- Treatment involves
  - ABCs
  - IV fluid replacement
  - Serum cortisol levels
  - Cortisol replacement
  - Vasopressors as needed

Bibliography

Budassi Sheehy S: Emergency Nursing Principles and Practice, 3rd ed. St. Louis, Mosby–Year Book, 1992.

Emergency Nurses Association: Emergency Nursing Core Curriculum, 4th ed. Philadelphia, WB Saunders, 1994.

Selfridge-Thomas J: Manual of Emergency Nursing. Philadelphia, WB Saunders, 1995.

Shlaffer M, Marieb E: The Nurse, Pharmacology, and Drug Therapy. Redwood City, CA, Addison-Wesley, 1989.

Chapter 6
Environmental Emergencies

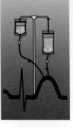

BURNS

Sources of Burn

- Thermal
  - Flame
  - Hot liquid
  - Hot grease
  - Hot metal
- Electrical: extent of injury determined by
  - Source of current (AC or DC)
  - Voltage
  - Path of current through body
  - Occurrence of arc
  - Type of grounding
  - High-risk electrical burn lesion:
    - Left arm: may indicate myocardial damage
    - Head: may indicate damage to brain, spinal cord, or ocular lens
- Chemical
  - Causes
    - Strong alkalis or acids
    - Alkali burns are more serious
  - Extent of injury determined by
    - Mechanism of action of chemical
    - Duration of contact
    - Inhalation
    - Surface area exposed

- Special considerations
  - Do not initially look for antidote, immediately flush with copious amounts of water
  - Remove all clothing in contact with chemical
  - Brush away solid chemical
- Lime: Brush away dry lime before washing lesions.
- Strong acids: If pain persists after initial flushing, apply a solution of sodium bicarbonate, magnesium hydroxide, or common soap.
- Strong alkalis: Continuously flush area for prolonged period of time.
- Phosphorus
  - Halt combustion by immersion in water.
  - Apply 1% copper sulfate solution to identify phosphorus particles.
- Hydrofluoric acid
  - Flush with copious amounts of water.
  - Subcutaneous injection of calcium gluconate may decrease tissue loss and control pain.

Depth of Burn

- Partial thickness (first- and second-degree burns)
- Full thickness (third-degree burns)
- Epidermal (first layer of skin only)
  - Erythematous, dry, blanches with pressure, painful
  - Example: mild sunburn
  - Heals in 3–5 days
- Partial thickness (first- and second-degree burns)
  - Superficial from epidermis to dermis
    - Blisters, edema, appears moist, bright red to pale ivory in color
    - Blanches with pressure
    - Heals in approximately 14 days

- Deep: from lower dermis to subcutaneous tissue (often seen with third-degree burns)
  - Mottled, waxy, dry or moist
  - Blistering and bullae
  - Takes several weeks to heal
- Full thickness (third-degree burns)
  - Through epidermis and dermis to subcutaneous tissue
  - May appear charred to pearly white, dry, leathery, inelastic, no blanching
  - Skin grafting usually necessary

Total Body Surface Area (TBSA)

- Palm estimation
  - An individual's palm represents approximately 1% of his or her TBSA
  - Useful for estimating scattered burns
- Rule of nines (see Fig. 6–1)
  - Adult and pediatric body is divided into multiples of 9 that total 100% TBSA
  - Useful in emergent assessment
- Modified Lund and Browder Chart (see Table 6–1)
  - Most accurate method to determine TBSA
  - Relates age of patient to body surface

Fluid Therapy

- Indications
  - Significant electrical burns
  - Partial-thickness or deeper burns
    - Greater than 20% TBSA in adults
    - Greater than 10% TBSA in children
    - Greater than 15% TBSA in elderly
- Objectives
  - Replace plasma volume

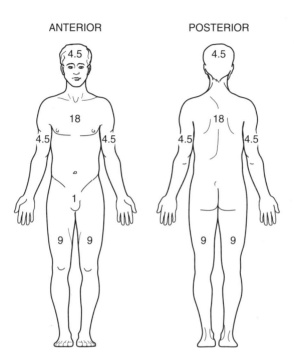

Figure 6–1. Rule of nines. The numbers represent a percentage of the total body surface area (TBSA).

- Maintain tissue perfusion
- Limit edema
- Initiate two large-bore IVs (use unburned areas if possible)
- Lactated Ringer's solution is fluid of choice because it is isotonic, similar to extracellular fluid
- Monitor glucose in children

Table 6-1. Modified Lund and Browder Chart

Burned Area	Age (years)					
	1	1 to 4	5 to 9	10 to 14	15	Adult
	Total Body Surface (%)					
Head	19	17	13	11	9	7
Neck	2	2	2	2	2	3
Anterior trunk	13	13	13	13	13	13
Posterior trunk	13	13	13	13	13	13
Right buttock	2.5	2.5	2.5	2.5	2.5	2.5
Left buttock	2.5	2.5	2.5	2.5	2.5	2.5
Genitalia	1	1	1	1	1	1

R.U. arm	4	4	4	4	4	4
L.U. arm	4	4	4	4	4	4
R.L. arm	3	3	3	3	3	3
L.L. arm	3	3	3	3	3	3
Right hand	2.5	2.5	2.5	2.5	2.5	2.5
Left hand	2.5	2.5	2.5	2.5	2.5	2.5
Right thigh	5.5	6.5	8	8.5	9	9.5
Left thigh	5.5	6.5	8	8.5	9	9.5
Right leg	5	5	5.5	6	6.5	7
Left leg	5	5	5.5	6	6.5	7
Right foot	3.5	3.5	3.5	3.5	3.5	3.5
Left foot	3.5	3.5	3.5	3.5	3.5	3.5

Adapted from the Emergency Nurses Association: Trauma Nursing Core Course Instructor Manual, 4th ed. Park Ridge, IL, Emergency Nurses Association, 1995, p 268, reprinted with permission.

- Fluid replacement is calculated from time of burn injury (see Table 6–2).
  - Up to 50% TBSA is considered. Replacement of fluids for more than 50% TBSA burn may result in overhydration.
  - For the first 24 hours:
    - Administer ½ total amount of fluid in first 8 hours
    - Administer ¼ total amount of fluid in second 8 hours
    - Administer ¼ total amount of fluid in third 8 hours
- Fluid resuscitation may be adequate if
  - Urine output is 30–50 mL/hr for adults, 1 mL/kg/hr for children
  - The patient is normothermic and normotensive
- Monitor for development of pulmonary edema
- Monitor vital signs

American Burn Association (ABA) Criteria for Burn Center Referral

- Partial-thickness and full-thickness burns greater than 10% TBSA in patients less than 10 years and more than 50 years of age
- Partial-thickness and full-thickness burns greater than 20% TBSA in other age groups
- Deep partial-thickness and full-thickness burns that threaten function or appearance
  - Face
  - Hands
  - Feet
  - Genitalia
  - Perineum
  - Major joints

Table 6-2. Guide to Determine the Rate of Fluid Replacement

Time	Solution	Parkland Formula	Brooke Formula
First 24 hours	Crystalloid	4 mL/kg/% burn	1.5 mL/kg/% burn
	Colloid	none	0.5 mL/kg/% burn
	Dextrose and water	none	2000 mL
Second 24 hours	Crystalloid	none	0.75–1.125 mL/kg/% burn
	Colloid	0–2000 mL	0.25–0.375 mL/kg/% burn
	Dextrose and water	2–4000 mL	2000 mL

- Full-thickness burns greater than 5% TBSA, any age
- Significant electrical burns (includes lightning injury)
- Chemical burns that threaten function or appearance
- Inhalation injury with burn injury
- Circumferential burns of extremity or chest
- Burn injury in patients with preexisting medical disorders
  - Diabetes
  - Alcoholism
  - Vascular insufficiency
  - Heart disease
- Burn injury with concomitant trauma

INHALATION INJURY

- Most common killer in fires
- Inhalation of smoke and other toxins leads to tracheobronchitis
- Inhalation of heat causes upper-airway damage
- Primary manifestation of smoke inhalation is pulmonary edema, which may not be evident for 24–48 hours
- High index of suspicion if the following are present
  - Facial burns
  - Singed nasal hairs
  - "Burning" discomfort in throat or chest
  - Carbonaceous sputum
- Important considerations
  - Length of exposure
  - Area of exposure (open versus enclosed space)
  - Type of material burned

Complications of Inhalation Injury

- Upper airway edema, hoarseness, stridor, dysphagia
- Atelectasis, tachypnea, hypoxemia, decreased PCO_2, dyspnea
- Interstitial edema, pulmonary crackles, tachycardia, cough productive of frothy pink sputum
- Bronchitis, frequent cough, dyspnea
- Pneumonia, fever, chills, cough productive of purulent sputum, chest pain
- Respiratory distress, increased respiratory effort, tachypnea, hypoxemia, elevated PCO_2
- Carbon monoxide poisoning
  - Carboxyhemoglobin levels greater than 10%, change in level of consciousness
  - Cherry red skin color, headache, dizziness, tachycardia, tachypnea, nausea

Initial Management for Inhalation Injury

- Establish patent airway
- Maintain nasotracheal or endotracheal intubation
- Ensure adequate breathing
- For moderate to severe burns provide the following
  - 100% humidified oxygen
  - Obtain arterial blood gases
  - Monitor pulse oximetry
  - Consider escharotomy for circumferential, full-thickness burns of neck, chest, or abdomen
  - Assisted or mechanical ventilation as required
- Ensure adequate circulation

- IV access immediately: preferred site unburned upper extremity
- Provide fluid replacement (see Table 6–2)
- Monitor patient response
- Frequent vital signs and reassessments
- Urinary catheterization necessary if more than 25% TBSA burn
- Urine pigmentation may indicate RBC damage, release of hemoglobin, muscle damage, release of myoglobin.
- Gastric intubation
  - For more than 10% full thickness burns
  - For more than 15% partial thickness burns
  - To decrease gastric distension from paralytic ileus
  - To prevent vomiting
  - To administer antacid
  - Secure with tracheostomy tape rather than adhesive tape
- Pain control
- Stop the burning process
  - Remove all clothing and jewelry
  - Cool water (never ice) soaks to burn areas
  - Maintain body temperature
- Administer IV analgesics and sedatives; avoid narcotics if patient has head injury
- Administer tetanus prophylaxis when indicated
- Obtain baseline laboratory tests
  - Complete blood count (CBC) with differential, electrolytes, glucose, blood urea nitrogen (BUN), creatinine
  - Carbon monoxide (CO) level
  - Blood type and screen
  - Clotting studies
  - Toxicology screen, as indicated
  - Urinalysis
  - Urine myoglobin and hemoglobin, as indicated

HEAT-RELATED EMERGENCIES

Heat Cramps

- Overworked, fatigued muscles (especially shoulders, thighs, calves, abdomen)
- Often associated with ingestion of large amounts of hypotonic fluids (water) during or after exertion
- Profuse sweating without salt replacement

SIGNS AND SYMPTOMS OF HEAT CRAMPS

- Muscle cramps
- Nausea
- Tachycardia
- Pallor
- Diaphoresis
- Cool skin

EMERGENCY MANAGEMENT OF HEAT CRAMPS

- Sodium chloride orally or intravenously
- Cool environment
- Rest

Heat Exhaustion

- Result of fluid and electrolyte depletion
- Often occurs over a prolonged period of time
- Especially in young and elderly
- May be associated with diarrhea or use of diuretics

SIGNS AND SYMPTOMS OF HEAT EXHAUSTION

- Thirst
- Malaise

- Muscle cramping
- Headache
- Nausea, vomiting
- Orthostatic hypotension
- Normal (or minimal elevation) body temperature

EMERGENCY MANAGEMENT OF
HEAT EXHAUSTION

- Fluids and electrolytes orally or intravenously
- Cool environment
- Rest

Heat Stroke

- Serious, may be life threatening
- Body unable to maintain normothermia
- Severe depletion of fluids and electrolytes
- Especially seen in elderly
- May be exercise induced in hot environment
- Increased core temperature
  - Depresses CNS, heart, and cellular function
  - Every 1°C (1.8°F) increase in core temperature results in a 13% increase in metabolism

SIGNS AND SYMPTOMS OF
HEAT STROKE

- Hot, dry skin
- Hyperpyrexia if more than 40°C (104°F)
- Tachycardia
- Tachypnea
- Hypotension
- Decreased level of consciousness

- Ensure ABCs
- IV fluid and electrolytes
- Rapid cooling measures
- Chlorpromazine (Thorazine) may be indicated to control shivering

COLD-RELATED EMERGENCIES

Frostbite

- Occurs in body parts exposed to prolonged freezing temperatures and wet environment
- Ice crystals form and expand in extracellular spaces if tissue temperature is less than 15°C (59°F)
  - Cell membranes rupture
  - Histamine release
  - Increased capillary membrane permeability
  - RBC aggregation
  - Microvascular occlusion
- Goal is to protect areas immediately surrounding the frostbite
- Often accompanied by hypothermia

SIGNS AND SYMPTOMS OF
SUPERFICIAL FROSTBITE

- Extends to subcutaneous tissue
- No blanching
- Tissue soft
- Usual sites: nose, ears, cheeks, toes, fingertips
- Burning, tingling, and numbness in area

EMERGENCY MANAGEMENT OF
SUPERFICIAL FROSTBITE

- Warm water soaks, maintain constant water temperature 40–43°C (104–110°F)
- Do not rub area
- Area will be painful, flushed, edematous after it thaws

SIGNS AND SYMPTOMS OF
DEEP FROSTBITE

- Extends to below subcutaneous tissue
- Tissue firm, unable to depress
- Previously frostbitten areas are at higher risk
- Skin is white, waxy
- Patient describes burning pain, warmth, then numbness with edema

EMERGENCY MANAGEMENT OF
DEEP FROSTBITE

- Prevent further heat loss
- Protect area from injury
- Apply warm water soaks, maintain constant temperature: 40–43°C (104–110°F)
- Provide warmed oral fluids
- Administer analgesics
- Consider tetanus prophylaxis
- Antibiotics may be indicated
- Escharotomy may be indicated in presence of vascular constriction
- After thawing, area may be bluish color, remain swollen, blisters may appear in one to seven days, and gangrene may develop later

Hypothermia (see Table 6–3, p.70)

- Core body temperature less than 35°C (95°F)
- Body is unable to maintain normothermia
- Contributing factors
  - Very young or elderly
  - Exposure
  - Health and nutritional status
  - Medications, drugs
  - Core temperature less than 28°C (82.4°F)
  - Pharmacologic and electrical interventions are usually not effective
  - Rewarming is the priority
  - Avoid discontinuation of resuscitation measures until core temperature is 32°C (90°F)
  - Avoid rewarming shock because
    - Peripheral areas are rewarmed faster than the core
    - Lactic acid is released and shunted to the heart

Bibliography

Budassi Sheehy S: Mosby's Manual of Emergency Care, 3rd ed. St. Louis, Mosby-Year Book, 1990.

Emergency Nurses Association: Emergency Nursing Core Curriculum, 4th ed. Philadelphia, WB Saunders, 1994.

Emergency Nurses Association: Trauma Nursing Core Course Instructor Manual. Park Ridge, IL, ENA, 1995.

Kitt S, Selfridge-Thomas J, Proehl J, Kaiser J: Emergency Nursing: A Physiologic and Clinical Perspective, 2nd ed. Philadelphia, WB Saunders, 1995.

University of Chicago Burn Unit Outreach Education Slides, August 1995.

Table 6-3. Manifestations and Management of Hypothermia

Category of Hypothermia	Temperature	Signs and Symptoms	Emergency Management
Mild	35–36°C 93–95°F	Conscious, alert Shivering, decreased Poor coordination Slurred speech Amnesia	Warm water bath 40–43°C (104–110°F) Glucose/sugars Avoid caffeine Warm PO fluids Warm blankets Warm environment
Moderate	30–34°C 86–93°F	Difficulty speaking No shivering Muscular rigidity Hyperglycemia Decrease in heart and respiratory rate and blood pressure Atrial arrhythmias	Ensure ABCs 100% O_2 Monitor pulse oximetry, ABGs Warmed crystalloid IV fluids (avoid lactated Ringer's solution) Monitor cardiac rhythm Monitor urine output Monitor core temperature

| Severe | <30°C
<86°F | Unconsciousness
Erratic, weak to absent pulse and heart tones
Significant hypotension
Erratic, shallow respirations to apnea
Ventricular dysrhythmias (ventricular fibrillation to asystole)
Cardiopulmonary arrest | Initiate active core rewarming
heated, humidified oxygen by mask or ventilator
warmed IV fluids 45°C
peritoneal, gastric, bladder or colonic lavage with warm fluids 45°C (113°F)
Hemodialysis or cardiopulmonary bypass (can increase core temperature 10–12°C/hr) |

Chapter 7
Emergencies of the Eye

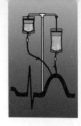

TERMS FOR DESCRIBING THE EYE

- OD = right eye
- OS = left eye
- OU = both eyes

EQUIPMENT AND PROCEDURES FOR EYE EXAMINATION

Wood's Light (Wood's filter, Wood's lamp)

- Light filter made of glass containing nickel oxide
- Transmits only ultraviolet rays
- Used to detect
  - Corneal abrasions after fluorescein stain
  - Fungal infections that fluoresce (i.e.: tinea capitis)
  - Presence of semen in a sexual assault examination

Slit Lamp

- Instrument with narrow beam, high-intensity light source
- Has microscope or binocular magnifier

- Used for visualization of the eye, especially anterior portions

Tonometer

- Instrument used to measure the tension of the eyeball
- Manually weighted (e.g., Schiøtz Tonometer)
- Computerized digital (e.g., Tonopen)

Fluorescein Stain

- Available in liquid, tape, and sticks
- A sodium derivative of resorcinolphthalein, $C_{20}H_{12}O_5$
- A fluorescing dye
- Used to diagnose corneal lesions and detect ocular foreign bodies
- Used in conjunction with a Wood's lamp

pH (paper, tape, sticks)

- Used to measure hydrogen-ion concentration of surface of eye contaminated with chemicals
- pH greater than 7 = alkalinity in an aqueous medium
- pH less than 7 = acidity in an aqueous medium
- Normal range for eye pH = (6.9–7.2)

Snellen Chart

- A chart for testing visual acuity
- Uses letters, pictures, numbers, or the letter "E" in various positions
- Wall mount or hand held

Visual Acuity

- A test of central vision
- Performed as a baseline prior to ED treatment for eye problems unless chemical burns or impaled objects, which are *true emergencies*
- Use a Snellen chart if possible

INTERPRETATION OF VISUAL ACUITY

- Position the patient 20 feet from the chart
- 20/20 vision = the patient can read at 20 feet what a person with normal vision can read at 20 feet
- 20/200 vision = the patient can read at 20 feet what a person with normal vision can read at 200 feet
- Test the visual acuity in each eye and then both eyes
- May be helpful to instruct patient to read chart in opposite direction with second eye to prevent memorization
- Test the visual acuity with and without correction (if applicable)

Detached Retina

- Vitreous separates or tears from the retina
- Fluid passes through a tear, lifts the retina off the back of the eye

SYMPTOMS OF DETACHED RETINA

- Flashing lights
- New floaters
- A gray curtain moving across the field of vision

*CONDITIONS INCREASING RISK OF
RETINAL DETACHMENT*

- Nearsightedness
- Previous cataract surgery
- Glaucoma
- Severe injury
- Previous retinal detachment in opposite eye
- Weak area in the retina

Glaucoma

- Leading cause of blindness
- Often asymptomatic in chronic open angle
- Loss of site is preventable with early treatment
- A disease of optic nerve
- Pressure in the eye increases when the drainage angle is blocked
- Increased pressure damages the optic nerve

TYPES OF GLAUCOMA

- Chronic open angle (most common)
  - Result of aging
  - Drainage angle becomes less efficient
- Narrow angle
  - Caused by a sudden increase in pressure
  - Width of the anterior chamber becomes critically narrow
- Angle closure
  - Complete blockage of the drainage angle
  - Rapid serious damage

*SYMPTOMS IN ACUTE ANGLE
CLOSURE*

- Blurred vision
- Severe eye pain

- Headache
- Rainbow halos around lights
- Nausea and vomiting

Central Retinal Artery Occlusion

- Sudden unilateral loss of vision
- Usually painless
- Caused by blockage of the central retinal artery by a thrombus or embolus

Irrigation

- Topical anesthetic (as prescribed)
- Minimum of 1 liter 0.9% normal saline
- Use of irrigation adjuncts (e.g., Morgan lens)
- Check initial pH and irrigate 10 minutes before rechecking pH
- Irrigate chemical burns until pH is within normal range (6.9–7.2)
- Caution patient not to rub eyes

Bibliography

Bates B. A Guide to Physical Examination, 3rd ed. Philade phia, JB Lippincott, 1995.
Gordon J: Instructional pamphlets for patients. James Gordon, MD. St. Louis, 1995.

Chapter 8
Genitourinary Emergencies

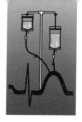

GENITOURINARY ILLNESSES AND INJURIES

Urinary Tract Infection (UTI)

- More frequent in females
- *Escherichia coli* is the most common pathogen
- Symptoms include
  - Burning
  - Frequency
  - Urgency
  - Hematuria
  - Malodorous urine
  - Systemic
    - Fever and chills
    - Nausea and vomiting
    - Malaise
- Abnormal urinalysis
  - Clean catch or catheterized specimen
  - Culture as indicated

Pyelonephritis (PYELO)

- Inflammation of the kidneys, including tubules, glomeruli, pelvis
- Can have same symptoms as UTI

- Generally the patient has a high fever and a much "sicker" presentation
- Flank pain

Renal Calculi

- Pain radiates from affected flank area to lower abdominal quadrants, groin, or legs
- Usually a dramatic presentation
  - Diaphoresis
  - Severe pain
  - Restlessness
  - Sudden onset of symptoms
  - Hematuria (gross or microscopic)
- Treatment
  - Fluids
  - Pain control
  - Radiographic studies (intravenous pyelography [IVP])
  - Possible surgical or lithotripsy intervention for large stones

Epididymitis

- An infection of the epididymis
- Signs and symptoms
  - Swelling and enlargement of the epididymis
  - Sudden tenderness of the spermatic cord
  - Fever
- Emergency interventions
  - Antibiotics
  - Rest with elevation of the scrotum

Testicular Torsion

- Twisting of the spermatic cord
- Signs and symptoms

- Severe scrotal pain and swelling
- Nausea and/or vomiting
- Fever
- Tense scrotal mass
- Emergency interventions
  - Ice to area
  - A true emergency to salvage the testicle
    - Manual manipulation
    - If unsuccessful, surgical intervention is necessary
  - Distinguish from epididymitis

SEXUALLY TRANSMITTED DISEASES (see Table 8–1)

GENITOURINARY TRAUMA

Urethral Trauma

- Blunt or penetrating trauma
- High degree of suspicion with pelvic fractures, perineal injury, penile injury
- Do not insert a catheter if injury is suspected or if blood is present at meatus

Ruptured Bladder

- Blunt or penetrating trauma
- Motor vehicle crash with "full bladder"
- Seat belt injury with "full bladder"

Kidney Trauma

- Blunt or penetrating trauma
- Can bleed into retroperitoneal space
- May have concurrent injuries (i.e., lumbar)

Table 8–1. Manifestations and Treatment for Sexually Transmitted Diseases

Disease	Incubation	Symptoms	Treatment	Comments
Neisseria gonorrhoeae	3–5 days	Yellow-brown purulent foul-smelling discharge; dysuria in men, may have a milky discharge from penis	Ceftriaxone "IM"	Also known as drip, whites, strain, GC
Chlamydia trachomatis	5–10 days	None to mucopurulent discharge	Doxycycline, tetracycline, erythromycin	Can be associated with GC

Organism	Duration	Symptoms	Treatment	Notes
Trichomonas vaginalis	7 days	Vaginal itch Frothy green-gray discharge	Metronidazole	Avoid alcohol
Gardnerella vaginalis	5–10 days	Frothy gray-white discharge that smells like fish	Metronidazole	Avoid alcohol
Herpes simplex II	2–12 days	Vesicular lesions Painful urination	Acyclovir	Latent and recurrent phases
Condyloma acuminatum	Days–months	Warty lesions, often asymptomatic	Topical podophyllin	May need surgical excision
Syphilis	3 weeks	Ulcer or chancre, + VDRL	Tetracycline, doxycycline, benzathine penicillin	

Common Treatment for Genitourinary Trauma

- ABCs (see Chapter 12)
- Fluids
- Appropriate radiographic studies
  - CT scan
  - IVP
  - Arteriography
- Treatment of concurrent injuries

Bibliography

Budassi Sheehy S: Emergency Nursing Principles and Practice, 3rd ed. St. Louis, Mosby–Year Book, 1992.

Emergency Nurses Association: Emergency Nursing Core Curriculum, 4th ed. Philadelphia, WB Saunders, 1994.

Fischbach F: A Manual of Laboratory Diagnostic Tests. Philadelphia, JB Lippincott, 1980.

Pagana K, Pagana T: Mosby's Diagnostic and Laboratory Test Reference. St. Louis, Mosby–Year Book, 1992.

Selfridge-Thomas J: Manual of Emergency Nursing. Philadelphia, WB Saunders, 1995.

Chapter 9

Selected Laboratory Tests

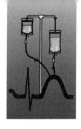

LABORATORY TESTS

- Lactic dehydrogenase (LDH)
  - Adult: 45–90 U/L
  - Child: 60–170 U/L
  - Infant: 100–250 U/L
  - Newborn: 160–450 U/L
  - In myocardial infarction (MI), LDH level rises within 24–72 hours. LDH peaks in 3–4 days and returns to normal in 14 days.
- Creatinine phosphokinase (CPK)
  - Adult Female: 30–135 U/L
  - Adult Male: 55–170 U/L
  - Newborn: 68–580 U/L
  - In MI, CPK levels rise 3–6 hours after infarction. CPK levels peak at 12–24 hours and return to normal 12–48 hours after infarction.
- Creatinine phosphokinase isoenzymes (CPK ISO): Enzymes may be fractionized to reflect specific tissue levels.
  - CPK-MM = 100%, specific for skeletal muscle
  - CPK-MB = 0%, specific for myocardial cells
  - CPK-BB = 0%, specific for brain and lung
- Coagulation studies (see Table 9–1)

Table 9–1. Coagulation Studies

Test	Normal Findings
Activated partial thromboplastin time (APTT)	30–40 seconds
Partial thromboplastin time (PTT)	60–70 seconds
Prothrombin time (PT)	11–12.5 seconds or 85–100%
International Normalized Ratio (INR) (corrects the PT ratios obtained by standardizing the results against a common international reference preparation)	2.0–3.5 considered to be the therapeutic range for patients receiving warfarin in the United States; can be a higher range in Europe with upper limits between 4.5 and 4.8
PT with patient on anticoagulant therapy	1.5–2x control value or 20–30%
Fibrinogen	160–360 mg/dL

LABORATORY TESTS RELATED TO HIV INFECTION

- CBC: Anemia is common.
- Platelets: Thrombocytopenia is seen.
  - Early because of idiopathic thrombocytopenic purpura
  - Late because of decreased production of platelets
- Differential: Leukopenia
- Chemistry: Impaired renal function
  - Elevated LDH
  - Elevated trigylcerides
  - Decreased vitamin B_{12}, B_6, and zinc
  - Decreased albumin levels
- Normal CD4 (T-4) range: 500–1500 cells/mL of blood
  - CD4 receptors are found on many cells in the body
  - CD4 count is the most useful clinical indicator of an HIV-infected person's immune system status
  - CD4 greater than 500 = low risk for AIDS-defining opportunistic infections
  - CD4 less than 500 but greater than 200 = low to moderate risk for opportunistic infection
  - CD4 less than 200 = AIDS by CD4 criteria; high risk for opportunistic infection

COMMON ELECTROLYTE IMBALANCES

Hypokalemia (Potassium Deficiency)

- Most frequent cause of potassium deficiency is through gastrointestinal loss

- Most frequent cause of potassium depletion is through diuretic therapy

CONDITIONS ASSOCIATED WITH HYPOKALEMIA

- Diarrhea
- Pyloric obstruction
- Starvation
- Malabsorption
- Severe vomiting
- Severe burns
- Primary aldosteronism
- Excessive ingestion of licorice
- Renal tubular acidosis
- Diuretic administration
- Liver disease with ascites
- Chronic stress
- Crash dieting without potassium supplement
- Chronic fever

SIGNS AND SYMPTOMS OF HYPOKALEMIA

- Cardiac arrhythmias (PVCs, atrial tachycardia, junctional tachycardia, ventricular tachycardia, ventricular fibrillation)
- Depressed T-waves, peaked P-waves on ECG
- Fatigue
- Muscle weakness or pain
- Paresthesia
- Hypotension and rapid pulse
- Respiratory muscle weakness
- Enhanced effect of digoxin

Hyperkalemia (Increased Potassium)

- Most frequent causes of hyperkalemia
  - Renal failure (inadequate excretion)
  - Cell damage (burns, trauma, surgery)
  - Acidosis (drives potassium out of the cells)

CONDITIONS ASSOCIATED WITH HYPERKALEMIA

- Addison's disease
- Renal failure
- Hypoaldosteronism
- Internal hemorrhage
- Uncontrolled diabetes
- Acidosis

SIGNS AND SYMPTOMS OF HYPERKALEMIA

- Muscle weakness
- Impaired muscle function
- Flaccid paralysis
- Tremors, twitching
- ECG changes (elevated T-wave, heart block, flattened P-wave)
- Cardiac arrhythmias (sinus bradycardia, sinus arrest, first degree AV block, junctional rhythm, idioventricular rhythm, ventricular tachycardia, ventricular fibrillation, asystole)

Hyponatremia (Decreased Sodium)

- This usually means excess body water rather than low total body sodium

*CONDITIONS ASSOCIATED WITH
HYPONATREMIA*

- Severe burns
- Severe diarrhea
- Vomiting
- Nonelectrolyte intravenous fluid in excess
- Addison's disease
- Severe nephritis
- Pyloric obstruction
- Malabsorption syndrome
- Diabetic ketoacidosis
- Diuretics
- Edema
- Water intoxication

*SIGNS AND SYMPTOMS OF
HYPONATREMIA*
- Weakness
- Confusion
- Lethargy
- Stupor
- Coma

Hypernatremia (Increased Sodium)

- This imbalance is uncommon.
- When it occurs it is associated with
  - Dehydration and insufficient water intake
  - Conn's syndrome (primary hyperaldosteronism)
  - Coma
  - Cushing's disease
  - Diabetes insipidus
  - Tracheobronchitis

- Dry mucous membranes
- Thirst
- Agitation
- Restlessness
- Hyperreflexia
- Mania
- Convulsions

Hypocalcemia (Reduced Blood Calcium)

- Conditions associated with hypocalcemia
  - Pseudohypocalcemia (reflection of reduced albumin)
  - Hypoparathyroidism
  - Chronic renal failure
  - Malabsorption
  - Acute pancreatitis
  - Alkalosis
  - Osteomalacia
  - Diarrhea
  - Rickets

Hypercalcemia (Excess Blood Calcium)

- Conditions associated with hypercalcemia
  - Hyperparathyroidism
  - Cancers that metastasize to the bone
  - Addison's disease
  - Hyperthyroidism
  - Prolonged immobilization
  - Excessive intake of vitamin D
  - Prolonged use of diuretics

Table 9–2. Criteria for Interpretation of Peritoneal Lavage in Blunt Abdominal Trauma and Penetrating Abdominal Stab Wounds

Positive	
Free aspiration blood*	
Grossly bloody lavage return	
RBCs	>100,000/mm³
WBCs	>500/mm³
RBCs†	>5,000/mm³
Negative	
RBCs	<50,000/mm³
WBCs	<100/mm³
Equivocal	
RBCs‡	50,000–100,000/mm³
WBCs	100–500/mm³

*Some investigators view any free blood as a positive result; others state that from 5 to 10 mL is necessary for surgical exploration.

†Criteria for interpretation of penetrating wounds to the abdomen and lower chest trauma.

‡50,000 to 100,000 RBCs/mm³ is an inconclusive lavage for blunt trauma and may be associated with a significant pathologic condition. Cases must be handled selectively.

RBC = red blood cell; WBC = white blood cell.

From Finis N: Abdominal trauma. In Kitt S, Selfridge-Thomas J, Proehl J, Kaiser J: Emergency Nursing: A Physiologic and Clinical Perspective. Philadelphia, WB Saunders, 1995.

- Respiratory acidosis
- Milk-alkali syndrome (excessive intake of milk and antacids)

Hyperglycemia and Hypoglycemia (see Chapter 5)

CEREBROSPINAL FLUID (CSF)

- Abnormal colors are due to
  - Blood
  - Bilirubin
  - Yellow pigments (xanthochromia) (previous bleed)
  - Dark yellow clots (subarachnoid block)
  - Protein more than 100 mg/dL results in an abnormal color
  - Carotenemia
  - Melanin (from meningeal melanosarcoma)
- Turbidity signifies
  - Increased leukocytes, especially neutrophils
  - Acute meningitis (slightly cloudy to pure pus)
  - Cryptococcal infection (turbid due to yeast cells)

PERITONEAL LAVAGE

- Associated conditions
  - Blunt abdominal trauma
  - Penetrating abdominal stab wounds
- Criteria (see Table 9–2)

Bibliography

Carmichael C, Carmichael J, Fische M: HIV AIDS Primary Care Handbook. Norwalk, CT, Appleton & Lange, 1995.

Dzung TL, Weibert R, Sevilaa B, et al: The international normalized ratio (INR) for monitoring warfarin therapy: Reliability and relation to other monitoring methods. Ann Intern Med 120:552–558, 1994.

Fischback F: A Manual of Laboratory Diagnostic Tests. Philadelphia, JB Lippincott, 1980.

Hirsch J, Poller L: The international normalized ratio. Arch Intern Med 154:282–288, 1994.

Kitt S, Selfridge-Thomas J, Proehl J, Kaiser J: Emergency Nursing: A Physiologic and Clinical Perspective, 2nd ed. Philadelphia, WB Saunders, 1995.

Pagana K, Pagana T: Mosby's Diagnostic and Laboratory Test Reference. St. Louis, Mosby–Year Book, 1992.

Chapter 10
Abuse and Neglect

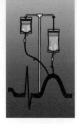

DOMESTIC VIOLENCE

- Physical or psychological abuse or assault
- Include a brief domestic violence assessment at triage
  - Does patient say injury was caused by another person?
  - Who?
  - Is story consistent with injury?
  - What is the patient's affect?
  - Is there a previous history of domestic violence episode(s)?
  - Are there other persons in the situation who may be at risk?
- Documentation of findings in the medical record is key
  - Photographs as needed to support documentation; check with your state's attorney to see if photography should be done by a trained expert
  - Diagram injuries on the medical record
- Report the event
  - Victim may not wish to press charges but have police interview the patient and make a report
  - Support the victim's decision
- Offer community resources
  - Does patient have someplace safe to go?

- Are necessary phone numbers, including assistance through 911, available (see Fig. 10–1)?
- Provide written referrals and community resources available

CHILD MALTREATMENT

- Physical, sexual, emotional abuse, and neglect
- Child abuse and neglect (real or suspected) is a mandated reportable event.

Causes of Child Abuse and Neglect

- Sociologic and environmental
- Parent stressors
- Child stressors
- Triggering situations
- History of abuse in the abuser

Signs and Symptoms of Child Abuse and Neglect

- Behavior of the child
- Behavior of the parent of caregiver

Shelter numbers _____

_____

Hot-line numbers _____

_____

Figure 10–1. Essential telephone numbers in the ED.

- Inconsistent story
- Ecchymosis
  - Various healing stages
  - Imprints of hands or objects
- New or old fractures inconsistent with mechanism of injury
- Abdominal injuries
- Burns
  - Thermal (spills versus immersion)
  - Cigarette (round, may look like impetigo)
- Head injury
  - "Shaken baby" syndrome
  - Retinal hemorrhages
  - Intracranial bleeds (see Chapter 14)
- Human bites
- Munchausen syndrome by proxy in which the caretaker
  - Keeps the child ill
  - Falsifies symptoms or history
  - Enjoys the medical attention given to the child

ELDER ABUSE AND NEGLECT

- Sources of abuse and neglect include
  - Family members
  - Institution
  - Hired caretakers
- Reportable event

Signs and Symptoms of Elder Abuse and Neglect

- Injuries inconsistent with a given history
- Ecchymotic areas in various stages of healing
- Marks around wrists or ankles from unnecessary restraint

- Patient may verbalize abuse
- Obvious signs of neglect
  - Alopecia or cradle cap
  - Severe dehydration
  - Signs of starvation
  - Deplorable hygiene
- Excessive sedation

EVIDENCE COLLECTION

- Chain of custody
  - Identify, label, and seal specimen
  - Prevent contamination of item
  - Assure specimen is from the source from which it is removed
  - Provide continuous tracking and possession of the specimen
- Preserve specimen as directed
  - Paper bag for clothing: Plastic prevents drying of clothing and promotes growth of mold, which may interfere with evidence.
  - Never cut through a bullet hole or stab hole in clothing.
  - Use a specimen container for bullets, glass, or small pieces of potential evidence.
- Label all bags or containers with patient's name, date, time, and signature and title of evidence collector.
- Secure all evidence in a locked area. Never leave evidence unattended.
- Include sexual assault collection kits.
- Place paper bags on hands of a suspected homicide victim to preserve evidence such as hair, blood, or skin that the victim may have on his or her hands or under the fingernails.

Bibliography

Bittner S, Newberger E: Pediatric understanding of child abuse and neglect. Pediatr Rev 2:197–207, 1981.

Budassi Sheehy S: Emergency Nursing Principles and Practice, 3rd ed. St. Louis, Mosby–Year Book, 1992.

Emergency Nurses Association: Emergency Nursing Core Curriculum, 4th ed. Philadelphia, WB Saunders, 1994.

Kitt S, Selfridge-Thomas J, Proehl J, Kaiser J: Emergency Nursing: A Physiologic and Clinical Perspective, 2nd ed. Philadelphia, WB Saunders, 1995.

Selfridge-Thomas J: Manual of Emergency Nursing. Philadelphia, WB Saunders, 1995.

Chapter 11
Medications

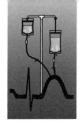

CONSCIOUS SEDATION

- Produced by administration of pharmacologic agents (see Table 11–1)
- Routes of administration may include IV, IM, epidural, sublingual, inhalation, and PO
- The patient under conscious sedation
  - Has a decreased level of consciousness
  - Maintains protective reflexes
  - Maintains patent airway independently
  - Responds appropriately to physical stimulation and/or verbal command
- Requires continuous monitoring during sedation until patient returns to presedation level: HR, BP, RR, pulse oximetry, and level of consciousness
- Emergency equipment: Drugs, airway and ventilatory equipment, defibrillator, and oxygen must be immediately accessible

DOSING INFORMATION

- Adenosine (Adenocard)
  - Give 6 mg bolus IV push (IVP) (2-second injection—antecubital/peripheral vein)
  - If given into an IV line, follow with a rapid saline flush
  - Observe ECG monitor for 1–2 minutes for conversion normal sinus rhythm (NSR)

Text continued on page 107

Table 11-1. Drugs Commonly Used for Conscious Sedation

Drug	Dosage	Actions	Nursing Considerations
Benzodiazepines Midazolam (Versed)	Dosage must be individualized and titrated Administer IV dose over 2 min Additional doses are in increments of 25% of initial dose after waiting an additional 2 min to evaluate sedative effect IV: adult: 0.1–0.15 mg/kg child: 0.035–0.15 mg/kg (max dose: 4 mg in child) PO: 0.3–0.8 mg/kg (max dose: 5 mg in child) Nasal: 0.2–0.5 mg/kg (max dose: 5 mg in child)	IV: Onset: 1–5 min Duration: 15–20 min PO: Onset: 30 min Peak: 40–60 min Duration: up to 3 hrs Nasal: Onset : 5 min Peak: 10 min Duration: 30–60 min	Depresses subcortical levels of CNS Rapid IV administration may lead to apnea Minimal analgesia Excellent hypnotic/sedative Excellent amnesia Used alone or with a narcotic Severe accumulation may occur in hepatic failure Transient apnea has been observed with dosages of 0.15 mg/kg IV Duration—slightly shorter than diazepam (Valium) Oral Versed: may need to flavor, use 5 mg/mL concentration Versed is 3–4 times as potent per mg as diazepam

98

	Rectal: 0.3–0.5 mg/kg	Rectal: Onset: 20–30 min Peak: 20 min	Dilute medication with 0.9 NaCl to a 1 mg/1 mL formulation to facilitate slower IV injection
	IM: 0.07–0.08 mg/kg (approx. 5 mg in adults)	IM: Onset: 15 min Peak: 30–60 min Duration: 2–6 hrs	
Diazepam (Valium)	Dosage should be titrated to desired sedative response IV: adults: 5–20 mg Do not exceed 2–5 mg/ min IVP MR with half dose q 5–10 min (max dose: 30 mg) IV: child: 0.2–0.3 mg/kg Do not exceed 1–2 mg/ min IVP MR q 15 min 2 mg/min MR with half dose q 5–10 min (max dose: 10 mg)	IV: Onset: 1–5 min Duration: 15 min	Depresses subcortical levels of CNS Also controls seizures Incompatible with all drugs in solution or syringe—do not dilute Caution in renal or hepatic disease Tablets may be crushed for oral administration Respiratory depression

Table continued on following page

99

Table 11-1. Drugs Commonly Used for Conscious Sedation (Continued)

Drug	Dosage	Actions	Nursing Considerations
Diazepam (Valium) (Continued)	PO: child: 0.2–0.5 mg/kg (max dose: 20 mg) PR: child: 0.5 mg/kg (max dose: 10 mg)	PO: Onset: 30 min Duration: 2–3 hrs PR: Onset: 10 min Duration: 1–2 hrs IM: Onset: 15–30 min Duration: 1–1½ hrs	Depresses subcortical levels of the CNS Caution in renal or hepatic disease Also used for seizures, anxiety, and other disorders Tablets may be crushed for oral administration Dilute medication with equal amount of compatible solution to facilitate slower IV injection
Lorazepam (Ativan)	IV: adult: 2–4 mg child: 0.02–0.05 mg/kg Slow IV push (2 mg/min) (max dose: 2 mg in child)	IV: Onset: 10 min Duration: up to 8 hrs	

Barbiturates
Thiopental (Sodium Pentothal)

IV: adult: 3–5 mg/kg
child: 2 mg/kg
Rectal suspension:
<3 mo: 15 mg/kg
MR after 15 min
7.5 mg/kg dose
child: 25 mg/kg
MR after 15 min
15 mg/kg dose
Neither children nor adults should receive more than initial and one repeated dose in a 24 hr period

IV: Onset: 30–40 sec
Duration: 5–30 min
Rectal: Onset: 3–5 min
Duration: variable
30+ min

Acts in reticular-activating system to produce anesthesia
Relatively long acting
Nausea is common side effect
Patient should be NPO 3 hours prior to rectal administration
No analgesic effects
Excellent hypnotic
May cause respiratory depression, bronchospasm

When using rectal suspension, adjust dosage downward to nearest 50 mg increment to allow for accurate measurement
Caution: cardiovascular, renal, liver disease, asthma, increased ICP
Table continued on following page

Table 11-1. Drugs Commonly Used for Conscious Sedation (Continued)

Drug	Dosage	Actions	Nursing Considerations
Opiates Morphine	IV: adult: 2.5–10 mg child: 0.1–0.2 mg/kg (max dose: 10 mg/ dose) IM: adult: 4–15 mg/kg child: 0.1–0.2 mg/kg (max dose: 15 mg/ dose) SQ: adult: 4–15 mg child: 0.1–0.2 mg/kg PO: adult: 10–30 mg	IV: Onset: 5–6 min Peak: 20 min Duration: 4–5 hrs IM: Peak: 30–60 min Duration: 4–5 hrs SQ: Onset: 15–30 min Peak: 50–90 min Duration: 4–5 hrs PO: Peak: 1 hr Duration: 4–5 hrs	Depress pain impulse transmission May cause respiratory depression Dilute medication with compatible solution to a 1 mg/1 mL formulation to facilitate slower IV injection Caution: bronchial asthma, increased intracranial pressure

| Fentanyl (Sublimaze) | Dosage is individualized
IV/IM: 1–3 µg/kg
Give IV slowly over 3–5 min
Total max dose = 4–5 mg/kg
Oral/transmucosal lollipop: 10–15 µg/kg
Begin use 20–40 min prior to onset of procedure | IV: Onset: immediate– 5 min
Peak: 3–5 min
Duration: 30–60 min
IM: Onset: 7–15 min
Peak: 30 min
Duration: 1–2 hrs
Transmucosal: Peak: 20–35 min
Duration: 1–2 hrs (erratic absorption) | Inhibits ascending pain pathway in CNS, increases pain threshold, alters pain perception
Potency is 100 times that of morphine
Both sedative and analgesic properties
Bradycardia and hypotension associated with rapid IVP or excessive dose
Mild respiratory depression, depressive effects 5 min after IVP, return to respiratory baseline in 30 min
Marked increased risk of respiratory depression with rapid IVP or excessive dose |

Table continued on following page

Table 11–1. Drugs Commonly Used for Conscious Sedation *(Continued)*

Drug	Dosage	Actions	Nursing Considerations
Fentanyl (Sublimaze) *(Continued)*			"Frozen chest," muscular rigidity, and masseter muscle spasm (difficult to ventilate) have been reported with rapid IVP or excessive dose May be used as a continuous infusion Less hypotensive effect than morphine or meperidine due to minimal or no histamine release Nausea and vomiting more frequently associated with lollipops Respiratory depression has been shown to last longer than analgesic effects

Miscellaneous			
Ketamine	IV: adult: 1–4.5 mg/kg child: 1–2 mg/kg (max dose: 100 mg given IVP over 1 min) Supplemental doses: 0.5 mg/kg IM: adult: 6.5–13 mg/kg child: 1–5 mg/kg (max dose: 50 mg) PO: 3–10 mg/kg Rectal: 5–10 mg/kg Nasal: 3–5 mg/kg Sublingual: 3–5 mg/kg	IV: Onset: immediate Peak: 1 min Duration: 15 min IM: Onset: 30–60 min Duration: 1 hr PO: Onset: 30 min Duration: 2 hrs	Phencyclidine derivative Acts on limbic system, cortex to provide anesthesia Less respiratory depression, except in large doses Sedation, analgesic, and amnesic effects Trance-like state, catalepsy, nystagmus Increased secretions Increased HR, BP Emergence unpleasant: vivid dreams, hallucination, increased frequency of dreams, hallucinations in adults May give atropine 0.01 mg/kg to children 10 min prior to administration of Ketamine Contraindicated in elevated ICP–avoid use with head-injured patient Dilute in equal amount of compatible solution to facilitate slow IV injection

Table continued on following page

Table 11-1. Drugs Commonly Used for Conscious Sedation (Continued)

Drug	Dosage	Actions	Nursing Considerations
Reversal Agents			
Flumazenil (Romazicon)	IV: adult: 0.2 mg IV initially given over 15 sec MR q 1 min (max dose: 3-5 mg in 1 hr) child: 5-10 μg/kg/dose given over 15 sec MR q 1 min (max dose: 1-3 mg in 1 hr)	IV: Onset: 1-2 min Peak: 6-10 min Duration: 30+ min Resedation may occur within 1 hr	Benzodiazepine receptor antagonist Reverses sedative effects of benzodiazepines Indicated with Versed, Valium Reversal effects of flumazenil may wear off before effects of benzodiazepine
Naloxone (Narcan)	IV: adult: 0.4-2 mg MR q 2-3 min child: 0.01-0.1 mg/kg/ dose May also be given IM, SQ, ET	IV: Onset: nearly immediate-2 min Duration: 30-40 min SQ, IM: Onset: 2-5 min	Narcotic antagonist Propoxyphene (Darvon) and pentazocine (Talwin) require very large doses to reverse Indicated with morphine, meperidine, fentanyl, propoxyphene, pentazocine Reverse effects of naloxone may wear off before effects of opiates

MR, may repeat.

- If paroxysmal supraventricular tachycardia (PSVT) persists, give 12 mg IV bolus, follow with a rapid saline flush
- If required, a second 12 mg bolus may be given
- Alteplase (Activase®) (see Table 11–2)
  - 3-Hour infusion: Total dose = 100 mg over 3 hours
    - Reconstitute the alteplase
    - Give 60 mg in the first hour via infusion pump; 6–10 mg of the 60 mg is given as an IV bolus over 1–2 minutes
    - Give 20 mg over the second hour via infusion pump
    - Give 20 mg over the third hour via infusion pump
  - Accelerated regimen for patients weighing more than 67 kg (>147.5 lb): Total dose = 100 mg over 90 minutes
    - Reconstitute the alteplase
    - Give 15 mg IV bolus over 1–2 minutes
    - Give 50 mg over the next 30 minutes via infusion pump
    - Give 35 mg over the next 60 minutes via infusion pump
  - Accelerated regimen for patients weighing 67 kg or less (147.5 lb or less): Total dose = <100 mg over 90 minutes
    - Reconstitute the alteplase
    - Give 15 mg IV bolus over 1–2 minutes
    - Give 0.75 mg/kg over the next 30 minutes (not to exceed 50 mg)
    - Give 0.50 mg/kg over the next 60 minutes (not to exceed 35 mg)
- Amrinone (Inocor) (see Table 11–3)

Table 11–2. Alteplase (Activase): Dose by Weight for Patients Weighing ≤67 kg (≤147.5 lb)

Weight (kg)	41	42	43	44	45	46	47	48	49	50	51	52	53
Weight (lb)	90	92.5	94.5	97	99	101	103.5	105.5	108	110	112	114.5	116.5
Total dose (mg)	66.5	67.5	68.5	70	71.5	72.5	73.5	75	76.5	77.5	78.5	80	81.5
Bolus dose (mg)	15	15	15	15	15	15	15	15	15	15	15	15	15
Next 30 minutes													
Infusion dose (mg)	31	31.5	32	33	34	34.5	35	36	37	37.5	38	39	40
Infusion rate (mL/hr)	62	63	64	66	68	69	70	72	74	75	76	78	80
Volume to be infused (mL)	31	31.5	32	33	34	34.5	35	36	37	37.5	38	39	40
Next 60 minutes													
Infusion dose (mg)	20.5	21	21.5	22	22.5	23	23.5	24	24.5	25	25.5	26	26.5
Infusion rate (mL/hr)	20.5	21	21.5	22	22.5	23	23.5	24	24.5	25	25.5	26	26.5
Volume to be infused (mL)	20.5	21	21.5	22	22.5	23	23.5	24	24.5	25	25.5	26	26.5

Weight (kg)	54	55	56	57	58	59	60	61	62	63	64	65	66	67
Weight (lb)	119	121	123	125.5	127.5	130	132	134	136.5	138.5	141	143	145	147.5
Total dose (mg)	82.5	83.5	85	86.5	87.5	88.5	90	91.5	92.5	93.5	95	96.5	97.5	98.5
Bolus dose (mg)	15	15	15	15	15	15	15	15	15	15	15	15	15	15
Next 30 minutes														
Infusion dose (mg)	40.5	41	42	43	43.5	44	45	46	46.5	47	48	49	49.5	50
Infusion rate (mL/hr)	81	82	84	86	87	88	90	92	93	94	96	98	99	100
Volume to be infused (mL)	40.5	41	42	43	43.5	44	45	46	46.5	47	48	49	49.5	50
Next 60 minutes														
Infusion dose (mg)	27	27.5	28	28.5	29	29.5	30	30.5	31	31.5	32	32.5	33	33.5
Infusion rate (mL/hr)	27	27.5	28	28.5	29	29.5	30	30.5	31	31.5	32	32.5	33	33.5
Volume to be infused (mL)	27	27.5	28	28.5	29	29.5	30	30.5	31	31.5	32	32.5	33	33.5

Table 11–3. Dosages for Amrinone (Inocor)

Body Weight		5 mg/mL Loading Dose	Infusion Rates (mL/hr)		
			5.0 μg/ kg/min	7.5 μg/ kg/min	10.0 μg/ kg/min
lb	kg	.75 mg/kg			
66	30	4.5 mL	4	5	7
88	40	6 mL	5	7	10
110	50	7.5 mL	6	9	12
132	60	9 mL	7	11	14
154	70	10.5 mL	8	13	17
176	80	12 mL	10	14	19
198	90	13.5 mL	11	16	22
220	100	15 mL	12	18	24
242	110	16.5 mL	13	20	26
264	120	18 mL	14	22	29

- APSAC (Eminase)
  - Use the drug within 30 minutes of reconstitution
  - 30 units IVP over 2 to 5 minutes by isolated infusion line
- Diltiazem (Cardizem)
  - 0.25 mg/kg (20 mg) IV over 2 minutes followed 15 minutes later by 0.35 mg/kg (25 mg) IV over 2 minutes
  - In atrial fibrillation with a rapid ventricular response, diltiazem may be used as a maintenance infusion of 5–15 mg/hour
  - Diluent volume: 100 mL
  - Quantity injectable: 125 mg (25 mL)
  - Final concentration: 1.0 mg/mL
  - Administration
    - 10 mg/hour, 10 mL/hour
    - 15 mg/hour, 15 mL/hour
- Dobutamine (see Table 11–4)
- Dopamine (see Table 11–5)

110

Table 11–4. Dobutamine, mL/hr: 250 mg in 250 mL D5W = 1000 µg/mL

Body Weight		Desired Dose µg/kg/min							
		1	2.5	5	7.5	10	12.5	15	20
lb	kg					mL/hr			
99	45	3	7	14	20	27	34	41	54
110	50	3	8	15	23	30	39	45	60
121	55	3	9	17	25	33	41	50	65
132	60	4	9	18	27	35	45	54	72
143	65	4	10	20	29	39	49	59	78
154	70	4	11	21	32	42	53	63	84
165	75	5	11	23	34	45	56	68	90
176	80	5	12	24	36	48	60	73	95
187	85	5	13	26	38	51	64	77	102
198	90	5	14	27	41	54	68	81	108
208	95	6	14	29	43	57	71	86	114
220	100	6	15	30	45	60	75	90	120
231	105	6	16	32	47	63	79	95	126
242	110	7	17	33	50	66	83	99	132

Table 11–5. Dosages for Dopamine, μg/kg/min: 400 mg in 250 mL D5W = 1600 μg/mL

Body Weight

		mL/hr							
		5	10	15	20	25	30	35	40
					μg/kg/min				
lb	kg								
99	45	2.9	5.9	8.9	11.8	14.8	17.8	20.7	23.7
110	50	2.6	5.3	8	10.7	13.4	16	18.6	21.3
121	55	2.4	4.9	7.3	9.7	12.1	14.6	17	19.4
132	60	2.2	4.5	6.6	8.9	11.1	13.3	15.5	17.8
143	65	2	4.1	6.1	8.2	10.2	12.3	14.3	16.4
154	70	1.9	3.8	5.7	7.6	9.5	11.4	13.3	15.2
165	75	1.8	3.6	5.3	7.1	8.9	10.7	12.4	14.2
176	80	1.6	3.3	5	6.7	8.4	10	11.6	13.3
187	85	1.55	3.1	4.7	6.3	7.8	9.4	11	12.6
198	90	1.5	3	4.4	5.9	7.4	8.9	10.3	11.9
209	95	1.4	2.8	4.2	5.6	7	8.4	9.8	11.2
220	100	1.3	2.7	4	5.3	6.6	8	9.3	10.7
231	105	1.25	2.5	3.8	5.1	6.3	7.6	8.9	10.2
242	110	1.2	2.4	3.6	4.9	6	7.3	8.5	9.7

lb	kg				µg/kg/min				
99	45	26.6	29.6	32.6	35.6	41.5	47.4	53.3	59.3
110	50	24	26.7	29.3	32	37.3	42.7	48	53.3
121	55	21.8	24.2	26.6	29.1	34	38.8	43.6	48.5
132	60	20	22.2	24.4	26.7	31.1	35.6	40	44.5
143	65	18.4	20.5	22.5	24.6	28.7	32.8	36.9	41
154	70	17.1	19	20.9	22.9	26.7	30.5	34.3	38.1
165	75	16	17.8	19.5	21.3	24.9	28.4	32	35.6
176	80	15	16.7	18.3	20	23.3	26.7	30	33.3
187	85	14.1	15.7	17.2	18.8	22	25.1	28.2	31.4
198	90	13.3	14.8	16.3	17.8	20.7	23.7	26.7	29.6
209	95	12.6	14	15.4	16.8	19.6	22.5	25.3	28.1
220	100	12	13.3	14.6	16	18.7	21.3	24	26.7
231	105	11.4	12.7	13.9	15.2	17.8	20.3	22.9	25.4
242	110	10.9	12.1	13.3	14.6	17	19.4	21.8	24.3

- Epinephrine (Adrenalin) (see Table 11–6)
  - Epinephrine infusion: start at 1 μg/minute and titrate to desired response (2–10 μg/min).
  - To prepare infusion: mix 1 mg in 250 mL (4 μg/mL)
  - Concentration 4.0 μg/mL
- Nipride (Nitroprusside) (see Table 11–7)
- Nitroglycerine (see Table 11–8)

Table 11–6. Dosages for Epinephrine (Adrenaline)

Dose μg/min	Rate mL/hr	Dose μg/min	Rate mL/hr
.500	7.5	10.50	157.5
1.000	15.0	11.00	165.0
1.500	22.5	11.50	172.5
2.000	30.0	12.00	180.0
2.500	37.5	12.50	187.5
3.000	45.0	13.00	195.0
3.500	52.5	13.50	202.5
4.000	60.0	14.00	210.0
4.500	67.5	14.50	217.5
5.000	75.0	15.00	225.0
5.500	82.5	15.50	232.5
6.000	90.0	16.00	240.0
6.500	97.5	16.50	247.5
7.000	105.0	17.00	255.0
7.500	112.5	17.50	262.5
8.000	120.0	18.00	270.0
8.500	127.5	18.50	277.5
9.000	135.0	19.00	285.0
9.500	142.5	19.50	292.5
10.00	150.0	20.00	300.0

Table 11–7. Dosages for Nipride (Nitroprusside), mL/hr: 50 mg in 250 mL D5W = 200 µg/mL

Body Weight		Desired Dose µg/kg/min					
		0.5	1	2	3	4	5
lb	kg				mL/hr		
88	40	6	12	24	36	48	60
99	45	7	14	27	41	54	68
110	50	8	15	30	45	60	75
121	55	8	17	33	50	66	83
132	60	9	18	36	54	72	90
143	65	10	20	39	59	78	98
154	70	11	21	42	63	84	105
165	75	11	23	45	68	90	113
176	80	12	24	48	73	96	120
187	85	13	26	51	77	102	128
198	90	14	27	54	81	108	135
208	95	14	29	57	86	114	143
220	100	15	30	60	90	120	150
231	105	16	32	63	95	126	157
242	110	16	33	66	99	132	165

Table continued on following page

115

Table 11–7. Dosages for Nipride (Nitroprusside), mL/hr: 50 mg in 250 mL D5W = 200 µg/mL *(Continued)*

Body Weight		Desired Dose µg/kg/min				
		6	7	8	9	10
lb	kg			mL/hr		
88	40	72	84	96	108	120
99	45	81	95	108	122	135
110	50	90	105	120	135	150
121	55	99	116	132	148	165
132	60	108	126	144	162	180
143	65	117	137	156	176	195
154	70	126	147	168	189	210
165	75	135	158	180	203	225
176	80	144	168	192	216	240
187	85	153	179	204	230	255
198	90	162	189	216	243	270
208	95	171	200	228	256	285
220	100	180	210	240	270	300
231	105	189	220	252	283	315
242	110	198	231	264	297	330

*Note: If you double the concentration by adding 100 mg to 250 mL D5W, divide the milliliters per hour by 2.

Table 11–8. Dosages for Nitroglycerin: 50 mg in 250 mL D5W (glass or special bottle)

mL/hr	μg/min
1.5	5
3	10
4.5	15
6	20
9	30
12	40
15	50
18	60
21	70
24	80
27	90
30	100
33	110
36	120
39	130
42	140

- Streptokinase
  - 1.5 million units over 30 minutes via infusion pump
  - Usually mixed 1.5 million units in 100 mL of diluent
  - Hypotension, flushing, and/or anxiety may occur within minutes of administration
  - Consult your institution's procedure (some institutions give diphenhydramine and hydrocortisone prior to giving streptokinase)

Bibliography

Barken R, Rosen P: Emergency Pediatrics: A Guide to Ambulatory Care, 4th ed. St. Louis, Mosby–Year Book, 1994.

Flanagan Miller A: Conscious Sedation Nursing Perspectives and Responsibilities. From an Independent Study Module. Offering Sponsored by American Healthcare Institute. Silver Spring, MD, 1994.

Skidmore-Roth L: 1993 Mosby's Nursing Drug Reference. St. Louis, Mosby–Year Book, 1993.

Chapter 12
Multiple Trauma

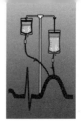

ABCs OF TRAUMA CARE

Primary Assessment

A = AIRWAY (PLUS SIMULTANEOUS CERVICAL SPINE IMMOBILIZATION)

- Assessment
  - Patency of airway
- Interventions
  - Suction
  - Remove loose foreign materials
  - Manual maneuvers: jaw thrust, chin lift
  - Airway adjuncts: nasal airway, oral airway, intubation (oral or nasal), surgical airway (see Chapter 18)
  - Stabilize cervical spine (hold in neutral position, apply rigid cervical collar, place head supports, and secure with tape)
  - Immobilize the spine (log roll onto long back board, secure with tape/straps)

B = BREATHING

- Assessment
  - Presence or absence of spontaneous respirations
  - Quality of respirations, rate, depth, effort, and use of accessory muscles

- Breath sounds
- Surface trauma, open chest wounds
- Interventions
  - Assist with bag-valve-mask as indicated
  - Assist with intubation (oral or nasal)
  - Supplemental high flow oxygen (non-rebreather at 12–15L/min) unless intubated, then 100%
  - Monitor SpO_2
  - Prepare for chest tube insertion with possible autotransfusion (see Chapter 18)

C = CIRCULATION

- Assessment
  - Quality of pulses (rate, distal, and central)
  - Skin signs (color, temperature, moisture)
  - Obvious external bleeding
  - Blood pressure
- Interventions
  - Direct pressure to external bleeding sites
  - Initiate two large bore (14 or 16 gauge) IV lines
  - Blood for baseline labs, STAT hemoglobin, hematocrit, glucose, type and cross match, toxicology screen, and so forth may be obtained with venipuncture for IV access
  - IV fluid of *warmed* lactated Ringers or 0.9% NaCl
  - CPR as indicated with advanced life support measures
  - Assist with thoracotomy as indicated

D = DISABILITY (BRIEF NEUROLOGIC ASSESSMENT)

- Assessment
  - Level of consciousness (AVPU = alert, verbal, pain, unresponsive)

- Pupillary assessment
- Interventions
  - Hyperventilation as indicated by focal neurologic signs
  - Glucose as indicated by documented hypoglycemia
  - Naloxone as indicated or in suspected narcotic use
  - Flumazenil as indicated or in suspected benzodiazepine use

Secondary Assessment

E = EXPOSURE

- Expose the patient completely
- Identify all injuries

F = FAHRENHEIT

- Maintain normothermia
- Prevent heat loss by use of overhead warmers, blankets, warm IV fluids

G = GET

- Get vital signs (temperature, blood pressure, heart rate, respiratory rate)

H^1 = HISTORY

- Mechanism of injury
- Treatment prior to arrival in ED
- Past medical history
- Medications
- Allergies
- Tetanus immunization status

H^2 = HEAD-TO-TOE ASSESSMENT

- Collect data by use of inspection, auscultation, palpation
- Consider congruence of history as it relates to possible child maltreatment, elder abuse, or domestic violence
- Perform systematic assessment from head to lower extremities, including posterior surfaces
- Determine revised Trauma score (see Fig. 12–1)

PENETRATING INJURIES

- Underlying tissues are damaged in the path of the wound.
- Wound may be caused by instrument or missile

REVISED TRAUMA SCORE

Respiratory Rate	10–29/minute	4	
	>29/minute	3	
	6–9/minute	2	
	1–5/minute	1	
	0	0	
			Total RR ____
Systolic Blood Pressure	>89 mm Hg	4	
	76–89 mm Hg	3	
	50–75 mm Hg	2	
	1–49 mm Hg	1	
	0	0	
			Total SBP ____
Glasgow Coma Points	13–15	4	
	9–12	3	
	6–8	2	
	4–5	1	
	3	0	
			Total GCS points ____

Total Revised Trauma Score _____

Figure 12–1. Determination of a revised trauma score.

Stab Wounds

- Length of the instrument
- Angle of the entry into tissue
- Velocity of stabbing force
- Gender of the assailant: men tend to stab with upward thrust; women attack with downward thrust
- Multiple body cavities can be penetrated by a single stab wound
- Damage to adjacent structures out of direct path of stab wound may be present resulting from disruption and displacement of tissue during injury

Firearm Injuries

- Projectile mass, shape, size, and composition
- Type of tissue penetrated
- Velocity of bullet (depends on distance)
  - Low-velocity missiles (<1000 feet/sec)(handguns) cause little cavitation or blast effect
  - Low-energy transfer to tissues
  - High-velocity missiles (>3000 feet/sec) (rifles) compress and accelerate tissue away from the bullet
  - Creates a cavity with negative pressure behind the missile
  - Debris contaminates the wound
  - High-energy transfer to tissues
- Density (the greater the tissue density/specific gravity, the more energy/damage to the tissue)

HEMORRHAGIC SHOCK

- Estimate fluid and blood loss based on initial presentation (see Table 12–1)

Table 12-1. Estimated Fluid and Blood Losses for 70 kg Male, Based on Patient's Initial Presentation*

	Class I	Class II	Class III	Class IV
Blood Loss (mL)	Up to 750	750–1500	1500–2000	>2000
Blood Loss (%BV)	Up to 15%	15–30%	30–40%	>40%
Pulse Rate	<100	>100	>120	>140
Blood Pressure	Normal	Normal	Decreased	Decreased
Pulse Pressure (mm Hg)	Normal or increased	Decreased	Decreased	Decreased
Respiratory Rate	14–20	20–30	30–40	>35
Urine Output (mL/hr)	>30	20–30	5–15	Negligible
CNS/Mental Status	Slightly anxious	Mildly anxious	Anxious and confused	Confused and lethargic
Fluid Replacement (3:1 Rule)	Crystalloid	Crystalloid	Crystalloid and blood	Crystalloid and blood

*The guidelines in this table are based on the "three-for-one" rule. This rule derives from the empiric observation that most patients in hemorrhagic shock require as much as 300 mL of electrolyte solution for each 100 mL of blood loss. Applied blindly, these guidelines can result in excessive or inadequate fluid administration. For example, a patient with a crush injury to the extremity may have hypotension out of proportion to the blood loss and require fluids in excess of the 3:1 guideline. In contrast, a patient whose ongoing blood loss is being replaced requires less than 3:1. The use of bolus therapy with careful monitoring of the patient's response can moderate these extremes.

From American College of Surgeons. Advanced Trauma Life Support Student Manual. American College of Surgeons, 1993, p. 86.

Bibliography

Cardona VD, Hurn PD, Bostnagel Mason PJ, et al: Trauma Nursing: From Resuscitation Through Rehabilitation. Philadelphia, WB Saunders, 1988.

Emergency Nurses Association: Emergency Nursing Pediatric Course Instructor Manual. Park Ridge, IL, ENA, 1993.

Emergency Nurses Association: Trauma Nursing Core Course Instructor Manual, 4th ed. Park Ridge, IL, ENA, 1995.

Sheahy S: Manual of Clinical Trauma Care. St. Louis, Mosby–Year Book, 1989.

Chapter 13
Musculoskeletal Emergencies

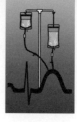

ASSESSMENT: THE FIVE Ps

- Pain
- Pulses
- Paresthesia
- Paralysis
- Pallor

SPRAINS AND STRAINS

Sprains

- Ligament is stretched until it tears
- Occurs when a joint exceeds its normal limits
- A more traumatic injury than a strain

Strains

- Involves muscles or tendons
- Occurs at the point where the muscle attaches to the tendon
- Caused by overstretching

Degree of Injury

- First = minor tear
- Second = partial tear
- Third = complete tear of ligament

Assessment of Sprains and Strains

- Distal circulation, motor, and sensation (CMS)
- CMS can also stand for color, movement, sensation
- Deformity, swelling
- Passive range of motion

Emergency Interventions for Sprains and Strains

- Immobilization with elastic bandage, rigid splint, or commercial product
- Crutches as indicated with gait training

RICE Mnemonic for Discharge Instructions

- R = **R**est
- I = **I**ce, application of cold
- C = **C**ompression bandage
- E = **E**levation of joint

DISLOCATION

- May be associated with damage to adjacent blood vessels and nerves
- Assess distal neurovascular status
- Determine the force/mechanism of injury
- Splint, immobilize the joint "as it lies" unless neurovascular compromise is present
- May be accompanied by fracture(s)

FRACTURES

Classification by Anatomic Location

- Distal
- Middle
- Proximal
- Intra-articular
- Head
- Shaft
- Base

Direction of Fracture Line

- Spiral
  - Fracture twists around shaft of bone
  - Results from a twisting force
- Transverse
  - Fracture is 90° to axis of bone
  - Results from angulation force or direct trauma
- Oblique
  - Fracture is 45° to axis of bone
  - Results from twisting force
- Comminuted
  - More than one fracture line and more than two fragments (includes segmental and butterfly fractures)
  - Results from severe direct trauma
- Greenstick
  - Incomplete fracture seen most commonly in children under 10 years of age; results from compression force
  - Impacted
    - One bony fragment is driven into another
    - Fracture line may not be clearly visible
    - Results from severe trauma

Blood Loss Associated With Common Fractures

- Pelvis: 750–4500 mL
- Femur: 500–3000 mL
- Humerus: 500–2000 mL
- Tibia/fibula: 250–2000 mL

Emergency Interventions for Fractures

- Immobilization with frequent assessment of distal neurovascular status
- Analgesics
- Closed reduction in the ED may require sedation (see Chapter 11)
- Surgical reduction may be necessary if unable to reduce in the ED
- Thorough discharge instructions

AMPUTATIONS

- Commonly associated with industrial or farm accidents and crush injuries
- Care of amputated part
  - Wrap the part in gauze minimally moistened with sterile saline
  - Place the wrapped part in a plastic bag and seal securely
  - Place the plastic bag in a container (or another bag) that has been filled with ice
  - Do not allow the part to freeze
  - Label with the patient's name
  - X-ray the part
- Care of the stump
  - Control excessive bleeding with direct pressure and elevation

- Clamping or ligation of the bleeding vessels is rarely needed
  - Avoid clamping or ligation if possible
  - Decreases the chance of successful reimplantation
- Avoid tourniquet use if possible. If used, note the time of application and the time of removal.
- Apply moist saline gauze over wound until reattachment or closure.
- Care of the patient
  - ABCs
  - IV access with fluid replacement
  - Maintain normothermia
  - Supplemental oxygen
  - Prophylaxis for infection (antibiotics)
  - Tetanus toxoid as indicated
  - Anticoagulation (aspirin per rectum) to increase chances of successful surgical reimplantation
  - Prepare for surgical closure or reattachment

COMPARTMENT SYNDROME

- An increase in pressure upon, or volume within, a fascial compartment of an extremity
- Compartments that can be affected
  - Shoulders
  - Upper arms
  - Hands
  - Pelvis
  - Hips
  - Thighs
  - Feet
  - Lower leg (2 compartments) and forearm (4 compartments) most commonly affected

Internal Factors Related to Compartment Syndrome

- Bleeding (note history of hemophilia)
- Edema

External Factors Related to Compartment Syndrome

- Constrictive bandages
- Casts

Classic Signs and Symptoms of Compartment Syndrome

- Throbbing pain
- Pain increases with passive muscle stretching
- Compartment pressures (see Table 13–1)

Emergency Interventions for Compartment Syndrome

- Remove external compressive force
- Elevate the limb *no higher than the level of the patient's heart*

Table 13–1. Compartment Pressures and Related Symptoms

Pressures	Symptoms
Above 30 mm Hg	Compartment taut, feels hard
	Skin blisters may develop
30–60 mm Hg	Muscle and nerve ischemia within the compartment
	Arterial flow preserved
>60 mm Hg	Arterial flow is occluded

- Administer analgesics
- Fasciotomy recommended when compartment pressures are between 30 and 60 mm Hg

SPLINTING

- Prevents further damage to nerves, blood vessels
- Decreases pain
- Splint above and below the site of injury
- Types of splints
  - Soft: pillows, slings
  - Rigid: boards, metal, cardboard, plastic, air, plaster, fiberglass, polymer
  - Traction: Thomas, Hare, Bucks; Hare used for femur fractures, proximal tibia fractures
- Angulation of extremity is corrected only if vascular compromise exists
- Application of cold packs is indicated in the first 24–48 hours
  - Apply for 20–30 minutes, every 2 hours
  - Elevate
- Use of pressurized ankle braces (e.g., Aircast)
  - For acute injury or chronic instability
  - Worn inside a sturdy shoe
  - Limits inversion/eversion of the ankle
  - Aircells and foam lining the brace provide graduated compression and allow for patient control of inflation and deflation
  - Massage compression contributes to the reduction of swelling and increased patient comfort
  - High altitude affects the expansion of the preinflated aircells
  - Velcro straps hold the rigid plastic splints in place
  - Weight bearing may be possible depending upon type of injury

Types of Splints

- Volar splint (see Fig. 13–1, p. 134)
- Boxer splint (see Fig. 13–2, p. 136)
- Thumb spica splint (see Fig. 13–3, p.138)
- Sugar-tong splint (see Fig. 13–4, p. 139)
- Posterior ankle splint (see Fig. 13–5, p. 142)

Bibliography

Aircast, Incorporated: Patient Fitting Instructions Insert. Summit, NJ, Aircast, Inc., 1990.

Budassi Sheehy S: Manual of Emergency Care, 3rd ed. St. Louis, CV Mosby, 1990.

Cardona V, et al: Trauma Nursing From Resuscitation Through Rehabilitation. Philadelphia, WB Saunders, 1988.

Emergency Nurses Association: Emergency Nursing Core Curriculum, 4th ed. Philadelphia, WB Saunders, 1994.

Emergency Nurses Association: Trauma Nursing Core Course Instructor Manaual, 4th ed. Park Ridge, IL, ENA, 1995.

Kitt S, Selfridge-Thomas J, Proehl J, Kaiser J: Emergency Nursing: A Physiologic and Clinical Perspective, 2nd ed. Philadelphia, WB Saunders, 1995.

1. Measure from 1 inch above the palmar crease to 2 inches from the antecubital. Prepare splint as directed.

Antecubital

2. Fold one edge of the splint over 1 inch. Place fold at the angle of the palmar crease (follow the life line).

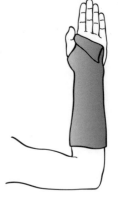

Figure 13–1. Volar splint. (From Ortho-Glass® Splinting Manual. Parker Medical Associates, Charlotte, NC, 1995.)

3. Wrap with elastic bandage to secure the splint. Mold and position as prescribed by physician.

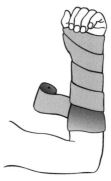

Figure 13–1 *Continued.*

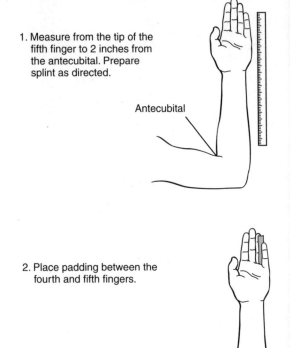

1. Measure from the tip of the fifth finger to 2 inches from the antecubital. Prepare splint as directed.

Antecubital

2. Place padding between the fourth and fifth fingers.

Figure 13–2. Boxer splint. (From Ortho-Glass® Splinting Manual. Parker Medical Associates, Charlotte, NC, 1995.)

3. Apply the splint to the ulnar side of the hand, creating a gutter.

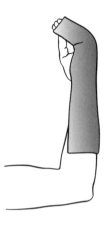

4. Wrap with elastic bandage to secure the splint. Mold and position as prescribed by physician.

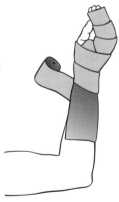

Figure 13–2 *Continued.*

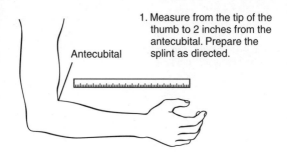

Antecubital

1. Measure from the tip of the thumb to 2 inches from the antecubital. Prepare the splint as directed.

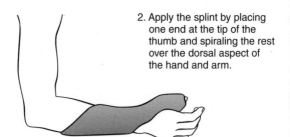

2. Apply the splint by placing one end at the tip of the thumb and spiraling the rest over the dorsal aspect of the hand and arm.

Figure 13–3. Thumb spica splint. (From Ortho-Glass® Splinting Manual. Parker Medical Associates, Charlotte, NC, 1995.)

3. Wrap by starting at the wrist and making two figure-eight wraps around the thumb.

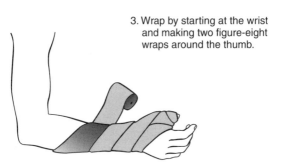

4. Mold and position as prescribed by physician.

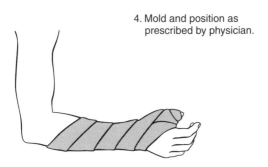

Figure 13–3 *Continued.*

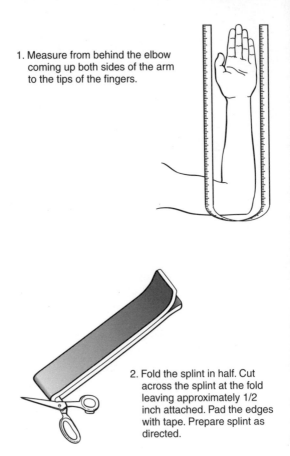

1. Measure from behind the elbow coming up both sides of the arm to the tips of the fingers.

2. Fold the splint in half. Cut across the splint at the fold leaving approximately 1/2 inch attached. Pad the edges with tape. Prepare splint as directed.

Figure 13–4. Reverse sugar-tong splint. (From Ortho-Glass® Splinting Manual. Parker Medical Associates, Charlotte, NC, 1995.)

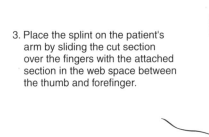

3. Place the splint on the patient's arm by sliding the cut section over the fingers with the attached section in the web space between the thumb and forefinger.

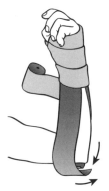

4. Wrap with elastic bandage to secure the splint. At the elbow, fold one side of the excess material behind the elbow and overlap with the other side. Lock in place with a series of figure-8 wraps.

Figure 13–4 *Continued.*

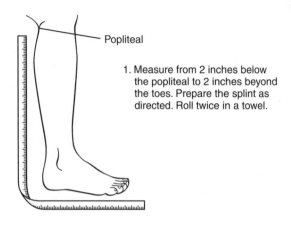

Popliteal

1. Measure from 2 inches below the popliteal to 2 inches beyond the toes. Prepare the splint as directed. Roll twice in a towel.

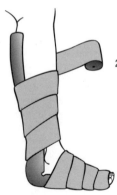

2. Fold the splint under 1 inch at the toes to make a reinforcing toe plate. Place the splint under the foot, extending slightly beyond the toes and wrap as follows: start at the toes, work up the foot, skip the ankle, and wrap behind the achilles.

Figure 13–5. Posterior ankle splint. (From Ortho-Glass® Splinting Manual. Parker Medical Associates, Charlotte, NC, 1995.)

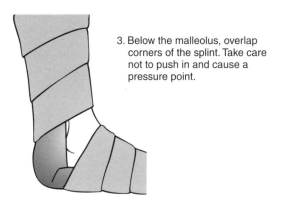

3. Below the malleolus, overlap corners of the splint. Take care not to push in and cause a pressure point.

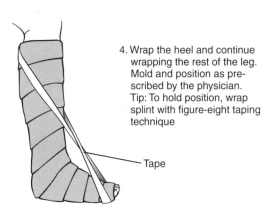

4. Wrap the heel and continue wrapping the rest of the leg. Mold and position as prescribed by the physician. Tip: To hold position, wrap splint with figure-eight taping technique

Tape

Figure 13–5 *Continued.*

Chapter 14
Neurologic Emergencies

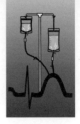

GLASGOW COMA SCALE (GCS)

- Reliable tool for evaluating level of consciousness
- Component of revised trauma score (see Fig. 14–1)

AVPU SCALE

- Provides rapid assessment of level of consciousness
- Does not rate or score the level of response
- Used when condition limits use of GCS
  - A = **A**lert
  - V = **V**erbal stimuli (response to)
  - P = **P**ainful stimuli (response to)
  - U = **U**nconscious

PUPILLARY CHANGES

- P = **P**upils
- E = **E**qual
- R = **R**ound
- R = **R**eactive
- L = (to) **L**ight
- A = **A**ccommodation

TEST	SCORE

Verbal Response

Oriented	5
Confused	4
Inappropriate words	3
Incomprehensible	2
None	1
Total	___

Eye Opening Response

Spontaneously	4
To speech	3
To pain	2
None	1
Total	___

Motor Response

Obeys	6
Localizes	5
Withdraws	4
Abnormal flexion	3
Abnormal extension	2
None	1
Total	___

Cumulative Total: _____ = Glasgow Coma Score

Figure 14–1. Scoring for the Glasgow Coma Scale.

EXTRAOCULAR MOVEMENTS (EOMs)

- Movement of eye controlled by coordinated action of six muscles (see Fig. 14–2)

145

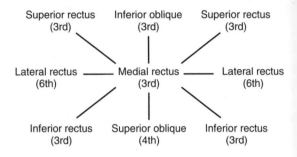

Figure 14–2. Six muscles controlling extraocular movement.

- Tests muscle function and nerve that supplies it
- Six directions of movement = cardinal fields of gaze

INCREASED INTRACRANIAL PRESSURE

- Increasing headache
- Increasing restlessness and decreasing level of consciousness
- Change in vital signs
  - Increased BP, decreased HR
  - Change in respiratory pattern
- Eye or pupillary changes
- Worsening of focal neurologic symptoms
- New onset of hemiplegia, hemiparesis, or hemianesthesia

DIAGNOSTIC PROCEDURES FOR NEUROLOGIC ASSESSMENT

- Doll's eye reflex
  - Do not perform if suspected cervical spine injury

- Place patient in supine position
- Examiner grasps patient's head and rotates only the head to the right, then returns to midline
- The patient's head is then rotated to the left and returned to midline
- Abnormal or absent doll's eye reflex
  - Head is rotated to the right or left, the eyes stay in midline or fixed in position
  - Structural and functional integrity of the brainstem may be affected
- A normal doll's eye reflex is observed when the patient's eyes move in a direction opposite of the direction the head is rotated
- Deep tendon reflexes (DTRs)
  - Abnormality may indicate pathology of
    - Cerebellum
    - Anterior horn cells
    - Peripheral nerves
  - Reflexes are scored 0 to 4+
    - 0 = absent
    - 1+ = decreased
    - 2+ = normal
    - 3+ = increased
    - 4+ = hyperactive

Tests to Identify Meningeal Irritation

- Positive Brudzinski's and Kernig's signs accompanied by
  - Fever
  - Headache
  - Chills
  - Nuchal rigidity
  - Indicates possible meningitis

- Brudzinski's sign
  - Place patient in a supine position
  - Examiner's hands are positioned behind the patient's neck
  - Gently bend the neck forward
  - Positive Brudzinski's sign
    - Presence of pain and resistance
    - Patient flexes hips and knees in response
- Kernig's Sign
  - Place patient in a supine position
  - Examiner first flexes patient's leg at the hip and knee
  - Try to straighten the patient's knee, leaving hip flexed
  - Positive Kernig's sign: Presence of pain and resistance

DERM Mnemonic (see Table 14–1)

Posturing

- Decorticate
  - Lesion of cerebral hemisphere
  - Flexion posturing
    - Unilateral or bilateral elbow, wrist, finger
    - Shoulder abduction and flexion
    - Plantar flexion of the feet
- Decerebrate
  - Lesion in the midbrain
  - Lesion in upper brain stem
    - Teeth clenched
    - Arms adducted, extended, hyperpronated
    - Legs extended
    - Plantar flexion of feet

Cranial Nerve Assessment (see Table 14–2)

Table 14-1. DERM Mnemonic for Assessment of Brain Stem Function

Herniation Levels	D — Depth of Coma	E — Eyes	R — Respiration	M — Motor Functioning	Positioning
None	Awake, alert, oriented	Equal and reactive	Eupnea	Normal	None
Thalamus	Painful stimulus causes nonpurposeful response	Small, react to light	Cheyne-Stokes respirations	Hyperactive deep tendon reflexes	Abnormal flexion (decorticate)
Midbrain	Painful stimulus causes no response	Midpoint to dilated; fixed; no reaction to light	Central neurogenic breathing	Decreased deep tendon reflexes	Abnormal extension (decerebrate)
Pons and Cerebellum	Painful stimulus causes no response	Pinpoint; fixed; no reaction to light	Biot's respirations	Flaccid	No tone
Medulla	Painful stimulus causes no response	Midpoint to dilated; fixed; no reaction to light	Ataxia; apneusis	Flaccid	No tone

Used with permission from Budassi Sheehy S: Emergency Nursing Principles and Practice, 3rd ed. St. Louis, Mosby–Year Book, 1992.

149

Table 14–2. Cranial Nerves and Related Mnemonic

Cranial Nerves	Mnemonic
Olfactory (I)	ON
Optic (II)	OLD
Oculomotor (III)	OLYMPUS
Trochlear (IV)	TOWERING
Trigeminal (V)	TOPS
Abducens (VI)	A
Facial (VII)	FINN
Acoustic (VIII)	AND
Glossopharyngeal (IX)	GERMAN
Vagus (X)	VIEWED
Spinal Accessory (XI)	SOME
Hypoglossal (XII)	HOPS

Mnemonics for Patients with Coma of Unknown Etiology

- AEIOU TIPS
  - A = **A**lcohol
  - E = **E**ncephalopathy / endocrinopathy / electrolytes
  - I = **I**nsulin / **I**ntussusception
  - O = **O**piates
  - U = **U**remia
  - T = **T**rauma
  - I = **I**nfection
  - P = **P**sychiatric
  - S = **S**eizure

- I SPOUT A VEIN
  - I = **I**nsulin (too much, too little)
  - S = **S**hock

- P = **P**sychogenic
- O = **O**piates and other drugs
- U = **U**remia and other metabolic abnormalities
- T = **T**rauma
- A = **A**lcohol
- V = **V**ascular
- E = **E**ncephalopathy
- I = **I**nfection
- N = **N**eoplasm

SEIZURES

- Abnormal electrical activity in the brain
- Seizures are a symptom, not a diagnosis

Types of Seizures

- Partial (seizure activity usually limited to one specific body part)
- Generalized
  - Petit mal (absence)
  - Grand mal (tonic-clonic)
  - Myoclonic (single jerk of one or more muscle group)
  - Atonic (drop attack — sudden loss of muscle tone)
  - Akinetic (loss of movement without atonia)
- Unclassified: seizures that do not fall into the above categories
- Status Epilepticus
  - Series of consecutive seizures
  - Continuous seizure that has not responded to therapy

Stages of a Grand Mal Seizure

- Prodrome
- Aura (not all patients have an aura)

- Loss of consciousness
- Tonic phase
- Clonic phase
- Postictal phase

Treatment for a Grand Mal Seizure

- Protect the patient from further injury
- Loosen clothing
- Do not try to restrain the patient
- Do not force objects into the mouth
- Treat the cause

Conditions that Contribute to Seizures

- Seizure disorders
- Medication noncompliance
- Neurotrauma
- Fever
- Alcohol withdrawal
- Detoxification of abused substances
- Cerebrovascular accident (CVA)
- Pregnancy-induced hypertension
- Metabolic disorders

CRANIAL BLEEDS

Intracranial Bleed

- Occurs in 30–50% of patients with severe head injuries
- Symptoms of increased intracranial pressure (See previous section on signs of intracranial pressure
- Possible herniation of temporal lobe through the tentorial notch

- Sinuses can accommodate approximately 75 mL of fluid

Epidural Hematoma

- Bleeding between skull and dura mater
- Caused by traumatic direct blow to the head
- Usually has accompanying skull fracture
- May have a middle meningeal artery tear
- Characterized by short loss of consciousness, a lucid period
- May have dilated pupil ipsilateral to side of injury

Acute Subdural Hematoma

- Bleeding between the dura mater and the arachnoid membrane
- Usually result of an acceleration or deceleration injury
- Laceration of a vein where it crosses the subdural space

Chronic Subdural Hematoma

- May occur 4–8 weeks after a traumatic head injury
- May occur without trauma in elderly or patients with chronic alcoholism
- Symptoms can be confused with those of senile dementia

Subarachnoid Hematoma

- Bleeding between the arachnoid membrane and the pia mater
- Usually caused by rupture of a congenital aneurysm

- Also may result from hypertension or severe head trauma
- May exhibit signs of a metabolic coma
- May have respiratory difficulty

SPINAL IMMOBILIZATION

- The vertebral column is aligned at all times
- Cervical collars do not provide adequate cervical (C)-spine immobilization when used alone
- Head and body must also be immobilized in alignment (not only the C-spine)
- Immobilize all head-injured patients
- Immobilize all unresponsive trauma patients
- All patients will remain immobilized until C-spine has been definitely cleared
- C-spine x-rays must include all seven cervical vertebrae and T-1
- Absence of a fracture on initial C-spine x-rays does not definitively rule out spinal cord injury

- **SCIWORA: S**pinal **C**ord **I**njury **W**ithout **R**adiographic **A**bnormality
  - Most commonly seen in children
  - Paresthesia may be the only clinical finding

  - **SCIWORA** results from deformity of the intervertebral segments, which is self-reducing

SPINAL CORD INJURY ASSESSMENT

Sensory Dermatomes (see Fig. 14–3)

- Useful in assessment of injuries to spinal cord or nerve roots

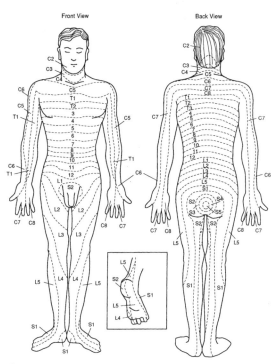

Figure 14–3. Dermatomes. (From Cardona V, Hurn PD, Bastnagel Mason PJ, et al: Trauma Nursing: From Resuscitation Through Rehabilitation, 2nd ed. Philadelphia, WB Saunders, 1994, p. 444.)

- Dorsal root of each nerve innervates sensation in a body portion known as a dermatome
- Examination is by pin prick and light touch to each dermatome

Myotomes

- Distribution of motor activity in body portions
- Tests for integrity of corticospinal tracts (see Table 14–3)

Table 14–3. Tests for Corticospinal Function

Spinal Cord Level	Patient Performance	Muscle
C-4		Diaphragm
C-5	Raise arms	Deltoid
C-5, C-6	Flex elbows	Biceps
C-6	Extend wrists	Wrist extensors
C-7	Extend elbows	Triceps
C-8	Flex fingers	Flexor digitorum profundus
T-1	Spread fingers	Hand intrinsics
T-1 to L-2	Full vital capacity	Intercostals
L-2	Flex hips	Iliopsoas
L-3	Extend knees	Quadriceps
L-4	Dorsiflex feet	Tibialis anterior
L-5	Extend great toes	Extensor hallocis longus
S-1	Plantar flex ankles	Gastrocnemius
S-2 to S-5	Control of sphincter	Perineal sphincter

Bibliography

Bartin R, Rosen P: Emergency Pediatrics: A Guide to Ambulatory Care, 4th ed. St. Louis, Mosby–Year Book, 1994.

Bater B: A Guide to Physical Examination, 3rd ed. Philadelphia, JB Lippincott, 1983.

Budassi Sheehy S: Emergency Nursing Principles and Practice, 3rd ed. St. Louis, Mosby–Year Book, 1992.

Cardona V, Hurn PD, Bastnagel Maston PJ (eds): Trauma Nursing From Resuscitation Through Rehabilitation, 2nd ed. Philadelphia, 2nd ed. WB Saunders, 1994.

Emergency Nurses Association: Trauma Nursing Care Course Instructor Manual, 4th ed. Park Ridge, IL, ENA, 1995.

Gottlieb AJ, et al: The Whole Internist Catalogue. Philadelphia, WB Saunders, 1980.

Kitt S, Selfridge-Thomas J, Proehl J, Kaiser J: Emergency Nursing: A Physiologic and Clinical Perspective, 2nd ed. Philadelphia, WB Saunders, 1995.

Chapter 15
OB/GYN Emergencies

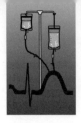

DEFINITIONS

- Gravida: Number of pregnancies, including the present
- Para: Number of pregnancies that have gone to at least 20 weeks' gestation, including stillborns

THIRD-TRIMESTER BLEEDING

Placenta Previa

- Partial or complete covering of cervical os by placenta
- Effacement and dilation begins
- Associated with multiparity, multiple pregnancy, breech, advanced maternal age

SIGNS AND SYMPTOMS OF PLACENTA PREVIA

- Sudden onset of painless bleeding
- Bright red blood from vagina

NURSING INTERVENTIONS FOR PLACENTA PREVIA

- ABCs
- Place patient on left side
- Give supplemental oxygen

- Provide IV access, crystalloid fluids
- Monitor fetal heart tones
- Prepare for emergency C-section
- Vaginal penetration or manipulation of the placenta (during a pelvic examination) may precipitate massive hemorrhage.
- No vaginal or pelvic examination is done until patient is in the OR with an emergency C-section set up

Abruptio Placentae

- Placenta separates from uterine wall prior to delivery
- Associated with hypertension, substance abuse, multiparity, precipitous delivery, trauma, short umbilical cord

SIGNS AND SYMPTOMS OF ABRUPTIO PLACENTAE

- Abdominal pain
- Contractions
- Uterine rigidity
- Presence of dark red vaginal bleeding
- Bleeding may be occult; assess for increasing fundal height

NURSING INTERVENTIONS FOR ABRUPTIO PLACENTAE

- ABCs
- Provide supplemental oxygen
- Provide IV access, crystalloid fluids
- Monitor fetal heart tones
- Mark and monitor fundal height on abdomen
- Prepare for emergency C-section

- No vaginal or pelvic examination is done until the patient is in the OR with an emergency C-section set up

FETAL HEART TONES (FHT)

- Most easily heard with Doppler stethoscope
- Documentation of FHT and site; a diagram of the abdomen with site of auscultated FHT may be used
- FHT parameters at more than 37 weeks' gestation:
  - Fetal tachycardia: greater than 160 bpm
  - Fetal bradycardia: less than 110 bpm
- Fetal heart rate will change before maternal vital signs; monitor FHT closely

EMERGENCY DELIVERY

- Emergent assessment of imminent delivery
  - Increased or heavy bloody show
  - Bulging membranes/crowning
  - If membranes have ruptured, note the color of fluid.
  - Mother states "the baby is coming"
- Questions to ask when faced with an imminent delivery: These three questions will alert you to the potential delivery of a neonate(s) requiring resuscitation.
  - "Are you pregnant with more than one baby?"
  - "Do you use, or have you used, drugs during this pregnancy?"
  - "How many weeks or months pregnant are you?"
- Emergency delivery
  - Attempt to maintain a sterile field in a private area as much as possible

- Maintain a controlled delivery of the fetus to decrease maternal and fetal trauma
- Instruct the mother to pant with contractions
- Place (gloved) hand on fetal head as it crowns with fingers spread and directed toward rectum; the elbow will be up
- Apply gentle firm downward pressure, allowing fetal head to deliver slowly
- Check for umbilical cord around neck
  - If present, slip cord over head and shoulders
  - Rarely will it be necessary to clamp the cord in two places and cut in between the clamps.
- Suction the infant's mouth, then nose, with bulb syringe
- Deliver the infant's anterior shoulder (guide head downward), then posterior shoulder (guide head upward)
- Allow the rest of infant to deliver (this happens very quickly)
- Note time of birth
- Hold infant horizontally and again suction mouth and nose
- Immediately dry and wrap the infant to maintain warmth
- Double clamp the umbilical cord and cut in between the clamps, allowing 6–10 inches of umbilical cord from infant to remain
- Allow mother to hold infant as soon as possible
- Perform Apgar scores at one and five minutes (see Chapter 17 for Apgar score and steps of neonatal resuscitation)
- Place identification band on mother and infant
- Transport to labor and delivery as soon as possible
  - Do not delay transport for delivery of placenta, which may take up to 30 minutes to deliver

- If placenta is delivered in ED, send to labor and delivery with the mother

PREGNANCY-INDUCED HYPERTENSION

- Chronic hypertension
- Chronic hypertension with superimposed pre-eclampsia
- Toxemia, a general term, refers to a classic triad after 20 weeks' gestation:
  - Edema
  - Hypertension
  - Proteinuria

Pre-eclampsia

- Acute elevation of BP greater than 140/90, more than 30 mm Hg elevation systolic BP, or more than 15 mm Hg elevation diastolic BP
- Proteinuria
- May or may not have edema

Eclampsia

- Seizures or coma in a patient with pre-eclampsia
- All organ systems affected
- Decreased glomerular filtration rate (GFR) and renal blood flow, oliguria
- Coagulopathy resulting in thrombocytopenia, hemolytic anemia
- Small hepatic hemorrhages, elevated liver enzymes, pain right upper quadrant
- CNS symptoms:
  - Visual disturbances
  - Headache, apprehension
  - Seizures

- Hyperreflexia
- Effect on fetus
  - Placental infarction (secondary to vasospasm)
  - Fetal hypoxia

Nursing Interventions for Severe Pre-eclampsia or Eclampsia

- More than 34 weeks with adequate fetal pulmonary maturity: delivery is definitive treatment
- Prepare patient for transfer to labor and delivery
- Administer magnesium sulfate
  - Affects transmission of acetylcholine at myoneural junction
  - Decreases incidence of seizures
  - Given as 4–6 gm loading dose in a 10% solution over 10 minutes
  - Maintenance dose 1–2 gm/hr IV
  - Excessive magnesium sulfate
    - Loss of deep tendon reflexes (DTRs)
    - Hypotension
    - Coma
    - Respiratory arrest
  - Antidote: 10% calcium gluconate, 10 mL should be available at bedside
  - Monitor DTRs, RR, HR, BP, LOC, FHTs
  - Monitor intake and output (I and O), assess breath sounds for crackles
  - Initiate seizure precautions
  - Minimize external stimuli
  - Prepare for transfer to labor and delivery
- Control hypertension
  - Hydralazine
  - Labetalol

- Nitroprusside may be associated with fetal cyanide toxicity

PELVIC EXAMINATION

- Have patient empty bladder before examination
- Supine lithotomy position (most common)
- Legs in stirrups
- Buttocks to edge of table or cart
- If a gyne bed, cart, or table is unavailable, place a covered bedpan, upside down, under the patient's buttocks. Stirrups are not necessary.
- Equipment
  - Light source
  - Vaginal speculum
  - Gloves
  - Lubricant
  - For Papanicolaou smear:
    - Spatula
    - Cytology brush
    - Glass slide(s)
    - Fixative
  - For other tests:
    - Culture medium or DNA probes for chlamydia, gonorrhea
    - Wet preps (slides, test tube) for trich or yeast

DILATATION AND CURETTAGE

- Cervical canal is widened with a dilator
- Uterine endometrium is scraped with a curette

Purpose

- Secure endometrial or endocervical tissue for sampling
- Control abnormal uterine bleeding

- Therapeutic measure for an incomplete abortion
- Usually performed in the operating room

ED Considerations

- Surgical consent form usually required
- Presurgical labs as ordered or required
- If performed in the ED, conscious sedation or other anesthesia may be used (see Conscious Sedation section in Chapter 11)

ULTRASONOGRAPHY

- Uses pulsed ultrasound waves
- Noninvasive or invasive (if vaginal probe used)

Procedure

- Transducer placed on abdomen or into the vagina
- Converts mechanical energy into electrical impulses
- Photograph or video of the amplified impulses used for diagnosis

ED Considerations

- Patient must have a full bladder
- If NPO, insert a foley catheter before examination
- Involves no ionizing radiation
- Takes less than 30 minutes to complete

ABORTION

- Interruption of pregnancy or expulsion of the contents of the pregnant uterus before the fetus is viable

Types of Abortion

- Spontaneous (miscarriage): most commonly occurs in the 5th – 12th weeks of gestation
- Threatened: cervix does not dilate, and spontaneous abortion may be prevented
- Inevitable: unpreventable, spontaneous abortion will occur
- Incomplete: some but not all of the tissue is passed
- Complete: fetus and all related tissue are passed

ED Considerations for Abortion

- Save all tissue for pathology examination
- For genetic studies, do *not* place the fetus or tissue in formalin, saline, or any other preservative
- Send to the laboratory immediately
- Notify laboratory personnel if the specimen is for *genetic study*
- Oxytocin may be ordered
- Prepare for possible surgical intervention, including consent and any ordered or required labs

RH DETERMINATION

- Presence or absence of Rh antigens determines the classification of Rh + or Rh −
- RhoGAM (Rh$_o$D)
  - Rh immunoglobulin
  - Prevents isoimmunization
  - Prevents further fetal hemolytic problems during subsequent pregnancies
  - Given IM after Rh determination screening
- Follow your institution's policy for administration
- Usual dosage: 300 μg IM

Bibliography

Budassi Sheehy S: Manual of Emergency Care, 3rd ed. St. Louis, CV Mosby, 1990.

Emergency Nurses Association: Emergency Nursing Care Curriculim, 4th ed. Philadelphia, WB Saunders, 1994.

Kitt S, Selfridge-Thomas J, Proehl J, Kaiser J: Emergency Nursing. A Physiologic and Clinical Perspective, 2nd ed. Philadelphia, WB Saunders, 1995.

Markovchick V, Pons P, Wolfe R: Emergency Medicine Secrets. Philadelphia, Hanley & Belfus, Inc., 1993.

Chapter 16

Organ Donation and Transplantation

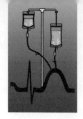

ORGAN DONOR CRITERIA

- Heart-beating donors (brain dead)
  - Age: newborn to 70 years (check criteria in your state)
  - Absence of sera + HIV or HBsAg
  - Organs: heart, lungs, liver, pancreas, small bowel, kidneys
  - Tissues: eyes, skin, bone, heart valves, saphenous veins
- Non–heart-beating donors
  - Age: 1–75 (check criteria in your state)
  - Absence of sera + HIV or HBsAg
  - Organs: none
  - Tissues: eyes, skin, bone, heart valves, saphenous veins

PRIORITY FOR CONSENT

- Next of kin
- Check criteria in your state
  - Spouse
  - Adult son or daughter (over age 18)
  - Parent (either)
  - Adult brother or sister
  - Legal guardian

ORGAN DONATION FLOWCHART

- Notify next of kin of death or imminent death
- Notify Procurement Agency of potential donor (see Fig. 16–1)
- Determine the suitability of the donor with the Procurement Agency
- Approach the family for discussion and request to donate tissue/organs
- Notify Medical Examiner as indicated by applicable laws in your state
- If donation is agreed upon, obtain order in chart for Procurement Agency to coordinate management of the patient
- Notify the operating room; obtain case start time (allow 3–6 hrs)
- Support the family, even if donation is not an option

ORGAN TRANSPLANT EMERGENCIES

Rejection

- Infection and allograft (a graft between individuals of the same species, but different genetic

---

Local Procurement Agency: _____

Phone: (_____) _____

United Network for Organ Sharing:

(800) 24-DONOR [(800) 243-6667]

Figure 16–1. Posted telephone numbers to facilitate organ donation.

makeup) rejection are the major causes of morbidity and mortality in transplant patients.

- Types of rejection
  - Hyperacute: Immediate rejection of the graft (usually while on the table)
  - Early acute: Rejection of the graft within 48–72 hours; sometimes reversible with OKT3 (monoclonal antibody that causes massive T-cell lysis)
  - Acute cellular: Most common from 5–10 postoperative days, but can occur anytime after 5 days after transplantation
  - Chronic: Usually untreatable
- Signs and symptoms of allograft rejection
  - Fever
  - Pain
  - Swelling or tenderness over the graft (especially if organ)
  - Possible weight gain
  - Shortness of breath
  - Nausea and/or vomiting

COMMON IMMUNOSUPPRESSANTS

- Cyclosporine
- Immuran
- Prednisone

COMMON ANTIREJECTION DRUGS

- OKT3: a pan–T-cell antigen
- MALG: antilymphoblast globulin
- ATGAM: antithymocyte globulin

INTERVENTIONS FOR TRANSPLANT REJECTION

- Rapid triage and placement
- History and symptoms of current illness (subjective)

- Transplant site and date of transplant
- Disease process leading to transplantation
- Previous history of rejection
- Physical assessment (objective findings)
- Complete vital signs including an actual weight if patient is able
- Inspection of the graft site
- Palpation of the graft site

Infection

- Some predisposing factors that increase the risk of infection in transplant recipients are
  - Diabetes mellitus
  - Prior hepatitis B and C
  - Leukopenia (reduction of the number of leukocytes in the blood <5000)
  - Splenectomy
  - Persistent uremia, azotemia, (an excess of urea, creatinine, and other end products of protein and amino acid metabolism)
  - Use of cadaveric donor organs
  - Repeated or persistent rejection treatment
- Bacterial infections are the most frequent infections in the solid organ transplant population and are usually associated with:
  - Technical procedures
  - Indwelling catheters
  - Other nosocomial exposures
  - Preexisting bacterial infections in the recipient
  - Bacteria present in the transplant organ

COMMON DIAGNOSTIC TESTS

- CBC
- Urinalysis
- BUN and Creatinine

- Liver function studies
- Drug levels (i.e., immunosuppressants)
- Pulse oximetry
- Electrocardiogram (ECG)

DRUGS THAT CAN INCREASE CYCLOSPORINE LEVELS

- Bromocriptine (Parlodel)
- Danazol (Danocrine)
- Diltiazem (Cardizem)
- Erythromycin
- Fluconazole (Diflucan)
- Itraconazole
- Ketoconazole (Nizoral)
- Metoclopramide (Reglan)
- Nicardipine (Cardene)
- Verapamil (Calan, Isoptin)

DRUGS THAT CAN DECREASE CYCLOSPORINE LEVELS

- Carbamazepine (Tegretol)
- Phenobarbital
- Phenytoin (Dilantin)
- Rifampin

Bibliography

Bromberg J, Grossman R: Care of the organ transplant recipient. Am Board Fam Prac 6:563–576, 1993.

Burdick J, Kittur D: Factors affecting early diagnosis of organ allograft rejection. Transplant Proc 23:2047–2051, 1991.

Nicholson V, Johnson P: Infectious complications in solid organ transplant recipients. Surg Clin North Am 74:1223–1245, 1994.

Chapter 17
Pediatric Emergencies

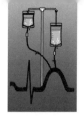

VITAL SIGNS IN CHILDREN (see Table 17–1)

MAINTENANCE IV FLUID RATES FOR CHILDREN

- 1–10 kg: 100 mL/kg/24 hr
- 10–20 kg: 1000 mL plus 50 mL/kg over 10 kg/24 hrs
- 21 kg or more: 1500 mL plus 20 mL/kg over 21 kg/24 hrs
- Example: 17kg child
  1000 mL + (50 mL/kg over 10 kg
  = 50 mL × 7 kg = 350 mL)
  = 1000 mL + 350 mL = 1350 mL
  = 1350 mL divided by 24 hrs
  = 56.25 mL/hr = maintenance IV fld rate

APGAR SCORE

- A standard rating system to describe the condition of a newborn.
- Assess at 1 minute and 5 minutes of age (see Table 17–2)

Table 17-1. Normal Vital Signs in Children

Age	Weight (kg)	Heart Rate (avg/min)	Respiratory Rate (avg/min)	BP (sys) (mm Hg)
Newborn	1	145	<40	42 ± 10
Newborn	2-3	125		60 ± 10
1 mo	4	120	24-35	80 ± 16
6 mo	7	130		89 ± 29
1 yr	10	125	20-30	96 ± 30
2-3 yrs	12-14	115		99 ± 25
4-5 yrs	16-18	100		99 ± 20
6-8 yrs	20-26	100	12-25	105 ± 13
10-12 yrs	32-42	75		112 ± 19
>14 yrs	>50	70	12-18	120 ± 20

Modified from Emergency Pediatrics: A Guide to Ambulatory Care. In Barkin R, Rosen P: Emergency Pediatrics: A Guide to Ambulatory Care, 4th ed. Mosby–Year Book, 1994.)

Table 17–2. Determination of Apgar Score

Sign	0	1	2
Heart rate	Absent	<100 beats/min	>100 beats/min
Respiratory effect	Absent	Slow, irregular	Good, crying
Muscle tone	Limp	Some flexion	Active motion
Reflex irritability	No response	Grimace	Cough or sneeze
Color	Blue or pale	Pink body with blue extremities	All pink

NEONATAL RESUSCITATION STEPS

- Assessment and resuscitation of neonate should occur simultaneously.
- Procedures performed most frequently are at the top of the pyramid in Figure 17–1. Most neonates require only the top level procedures (i.e., drying and warming).
- Resuscitation progresses step by step (rapidly) down the pyramid.

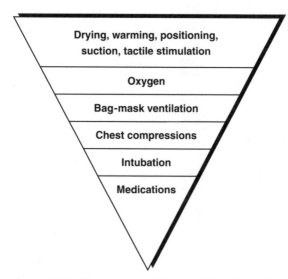

Figure 17–1. Steps in neonatal resuscitation. (From the Textbook of Neonatal Resuscitation. 1987, 1990, 1994. Reprinted with permission. Copyright © American Heart Association.)

- Evaluation of the neonate's response occurs (rapidly) between each step.

PEDIATRIC COMA SCALE

- A modification of Glasgow Coma Scale (GCS) by age (see Table 17–3)
- Score is the sum of the individual scores from eye opening, best verbal response, and best motor response
  - GCS of 13–15: mild head injury
  - GCS of 9–12: moderate head injury
  - GCS of less than 8: severe head injury

PEDIATRIC TRAUMA SCALE

- Useful as a triage tool
- Predictor of injury severity
- A score of $+2$, $+1$, or -1 is given to each variable, then added. Range: -6 to 12 (see Table 17–4)
- Score of less than or equal to 8 indicates potentially important trauma

ASSESSMENT OF DEHYDRATION (see Table 17–5)

- Decreased intake by mouth
- Excessive losses, vomiting, diarrhea
- Fever

ANTIPYRETICS AND ANALGESICS

Acetaminophen

- Dosage
  - 10–15 mg/kg/dose

Table 17-3. Pediatric Modification of Glasgow Coma Scale (GCS) by Age of Patient*

Glasgow Coma Score

Eye Opening

≥1 year
4 Spontaneously
3 To verbal command
2 To pain
1 No response

Best Motor Response

≥1 year
6 Obeys
5 Localizes pain
4 Flexion withdrawal
3 Flexion abnormal
  (decorticate)
2 Extension
  (decerebrate)
1 No response

Pediatric Modification

0–1 yr
4 Spontaneously
3 To shout
2 To pain
1 No response

0–1 yr

5 Localizes pain
4 Flexion withdrawal
3 Flexion abnormal
  (decorticate)
2 Extension
  (decerebrate)
1 No response

Best Verbal Response

>5 years	0–2 yrs	2–5 yrs
5 Oriented and converses	5 Cries appropriately, smiles, coos	5 Appropriate words and phrases
4 Disoriented and converses	4 Cries	4 Inappropriate words
3 Inappropriate words	3 Inappropriate crying/ screaming	3 Cries/screams
2 Incomprehensible sounds	2 Grunts	2 Grunts
1 No response	1 No response	1 No response

*Score is the sum of the individual scores from eye opening, best verbal response, and best motor response, using age-specific criteria. GCS of 13–15 indicates mild head injury. GCS of 9–12 indicates moderate head injury, and GCS <8 indicates severe head injury.

From Barkin R, Rosen P: Emergency Pediatrics: A Guide to Ambulatory Care, 4th ed. St. Louis, Mosby–Year Book, 1994, p. 385.

Table 17–4. Pediatric Trauma Score

Component	+2	+1	−1
Size	≥20 kg	10–20 kg	<10 kg
Airway	Normal	Maintainable	Unmaintainable
Systolic BP	≤90 mm Hg	90–50 mm Hg	<50 mm Hg
CNS	Awake	Obtunded/LOC	Coma/decerebrate
Open wound	None	Minor	Major/penetrating
Skeletal	None	Closed fracture	Open/multiple fractures

Sum total points

Reprinted with permission from Tepas JJ, Mollitt DL, Talbert JL, et al: The Pediatric Trauma Score as a predictor of injury severity in the injured child. J Pediatr Surg 22:14, 1987.

Table 17–5. Clinical and Ancillary Findings by Degree of Dehydration

Finding	Mild (<5%)	Moderate (10%)	Severe (15%)
		Signs and Symptoms	
Dry mucous membrane	±	+	+
Reduced skin turgor	−	±	+
Depressed anterior fontanelle	−	+	+
Sunken eyeballs	−	±	+
Hyperpnea	−	±	+
Hypotension (orthostatic)	−	+	+
Increased pulse	−	+	+
		Ancillary Data	
Urine			
Volume	Small	Oliguria	Oliguria/anuria
Specific gravity	<1.020	>1.030	>1.035
Blood			
BUN	Within normal limits	Elevated	Very high
pH (arterial)	7.40–7.30	7.30–7.00	<7.10

From Barkin R, Rosen P: Emergency Pediatrics: A Guide to Ambulatory Care, 4th ed. St. Louis, Mosby–Year Book, 1994.

- q 4–6 h PO
- Adult: 650 mg/dose
- How supplied
  - Drops: 80 mg/0.8 mL
  - Elixir: 160 mg/5 mL
  - Suspension: 160 mg/5 mL
  - Tablets, chewable: 80 mg
    - Junior: 160 mg
    - Regular: 325 mg
  - Suppository: 120 mg, 325 mg

Ibuprofen

- Dosage
  - 10 mg/kg/dose
  - q 4–6 h PO
  - Adult: 400–600 mg/dose
- How supplied
  - Suspension: 100 mg/5 mL
  - Tablets: 200 mg, 400 mg, 600 mg

AVERAGE GROWTH PATTERNS

- Newborns lose 10% birthweight initially but will regain loss by 10th day of life
- 5 months—double birthweight
- 12 months—triple birthweight, double birth length
- 2 years—quadruple birthweight

CHILD IMMUNIZATIONS

(see Table 17–6)

COMMON CHILDHOOD RASHES AND LESIONS

- See Table 17–7
- See also Chapter 3

Table 17–6. Recommended Childhood Immunization Schedule

Age	Vaccine
Birth	Hepatitis B*
2 mo	Hepatitis B, DTP, OPV, HIB
4 mo	DTP, OPV, HIB
6 mo	Hepatitis B, DTP, HIB, OPV (optional)
12 mo	TB test (optional)
15 mo	DTP, OPV, MMR, HIB
4–6 yrs	DTP, OPV, MMR
14–16 yrs	Td and thereafter every 10 yrs

*Hepatitis B vaccine may be given in either schedule: Birth, 1–2 mo, 6–18 mo, or 2 mo, 4 mo, 12–16 mo.

DTP = diphtheria, tetanus, and pertussis; OPV = oral polio vaccine; HIB = H. influenzae or *Haemophilus* b conjugate vaccine (HbOC is given at 2 mo, 4 mo, 6 mo, and 15 months; PRP-OMP is given at 2 months, 4 months, and 12 months); MMR = measles, mumps, and rubella; Td = tetanus and diphtheria.

Adapted from Centers for Disease Control: ACIP Recommended Immunization Schedule. Atlanta, GA, 1992.

INTRAMUSCULAR INJECTION

(see Fig. 17–2 and Table 17–8)

INTRAOSSEOUS INFUSION

Indications for Intraosseous Infusion

- Emergency administration of drugs, fluids, blood products
- Age 6 years or less
- Unable to achieve vascular access in three attempts or 90 seconds (whichever comes first)

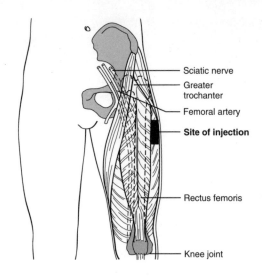

- Sciatic nerve
- Greater trochanter
- Femoral artery
- **Site of injection**
- Rectus femoris
- Knee joint

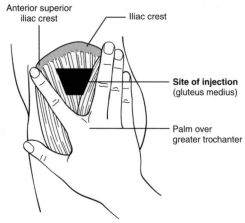

- Anterior superior iliac crest
- Iliac crest
- **Site of injection** (gluteus medius)
- Palm over greater trochanter

Figure 17–2 *See legend on opposite page*

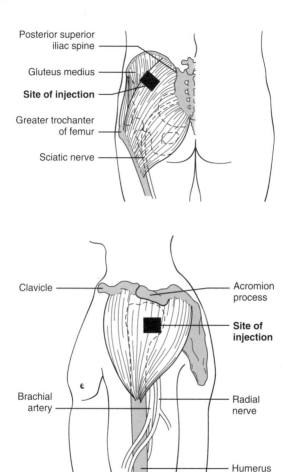

Figure 17–2. Intramuscular injection sites in children. (From Emergency Nurses Association: Emergency Nursing Pediatrics Course Instructor Manual. Park Ridge, IL, ENA, 1993.)

Table 17-7. Childhood Rashes and Lesions

Disease	Rash/Lesion
Chickenpox (Varicella zoster)	Begins as small red macules, progresses to papules, then vesicles; crusty lesions remain after vesicle ruptures; Pruritic; begins on trunk and spreads to face, and exits
Fifth Disease	Macular; on face, appears like "slapped cheeks"; lacy rash on arms, legs
Impetigo	Begins as vesicular lesions, then yellow crusts on red base; seen on feet, hands, face; pruritic
Kawasaki Syndrome	Begins as red maculopapular lesions, then confluent pruritic wheals; in 2–7 days, desquamation
Ringworm	Round or oval red scaly patches, central area clear; spreads outward
Roseola (baby measles)	Macules or maculopapular, small rose-pink; first appears on trunk; widely disseminated; no itching; preceded by fever
Rubella (German measles)	Maculopapular, pink/red; begins on head, spreads downward
Rubeola (measles)	Maculopapular, red; begins on face, spreads downward; confluent in 1–2 days; preceded by cough, runny nose, conjunctivitis, white lesions on buccal mucosa
Scarlet Fever	Maculopapular rash, fine ("sandpaper rash"), avoids facial area; red ("strawberry") tongue; red lines in axilla, antecubital area
Thrush (Candida)	White patches on mucous membranes, will not scrape off

Procedure for Intraosseous Infusion

- Localize insertion site (preferred site):
  - Flat, anteromedial surface of tibia
  - 1–3 cm below tibial tuberosity and just medial (may also use distal femur)
- Cleanse site, don gloves
- Using bone marrow needle, or specific I/O needle, insert needle at a 90 degree angle, or slightly toward toes to avoid growth plate. Use firm, twisting motion. Stabilization of child's leg is with your nondominant hand, being careful not to have hand behind insertion site.
- Withdraw stylet from the needle
- Attempt to aspirate bone marrow or flush with 5–10 mL normal saline through needle
- Assess resistance to injection, increased firmness of soft tissue
- Attach IV extension tubing (short length) to I/O needle
- Place IV stopcock between extension tubing and IV administration tubing
- Attach a pressure infusion device
  - Infusion by gravity is slow and inconsistent
  - Fluid boluses are administered by withdrawing IV solution into large syringe attached to stopcock, closing stopcock to IV bag, and depressing plunger of syringe, thus administering IV bolus of fluid
- Stabilize I/O needle with tape or gauze
- Continuously assess patency of I/O needle and check for extravasation of fluid, medication

Table 17–8. Pediatric Intramuscular Injection Site

Site	Recommended Age	Pros and Cons
Vastus lateralis (anterior lateral thigh)	Infant to adult Preferred for children <3 yrs	Largest muscle group in children <3 yrs Can tolerate large injection volumes (0.5–2.0 mL) Area free of important nerves or blood vessels
Ventrogluteal (lateral hip)	Infant to adult Consider for children >3 yrs	Can tolerate large injection volumes Area free of important nerves or blood vessels Easily accessible site

Dorsogluteal (upper outer buttock)	Contraindicated in children <3 yrs or in children who have not been walking for one year	Large muscle mass in older children Can tolerate large injection volumes Danger of injury to sciatic nerve Exposure of site may cause embarrassment in older child
Deltoid	Infant to adult	Small muscle mass Can tolerate only small injection volumes (0.5–1.0 mL) Easily accessible site Danger of radial nerve injury in young children

Adapted from Emergency Nurses Association: Emergency Nursing Pediatric Course Instructor Manual. Park Ridge, IL, ENA, 1993, used with permission.

PEDIATRIC LIFE SUPPORT

- The American Heart Association's Pediatric Basic Life Support Courses and Pediatric Advanced Life Support Courses are recommended for all ED nurses caring for children.

Pediatric Advanced Life Support

- The key is *early* recognition of the child in respiratory distress or "early" shock.
- Signs and symptoms of respiratory distress:
  - Increased respiratory effort (or decreased respiratory effort as child becomes fatigued)
  - Decreased respiratory rate
  - Poor chest excursion
  - Decreased breath sounds
  - Decreased LOC
  - Decreased muscle tone
  - Color change: pale, cyanosis
- Signs and symptoms of "early" shock:
  - Increased HR, or decreased HR as child fatigues, preterminal bradycardia rhythm
  - Poor-quality distal pulses or absence of distal pulses in presence of central pulses
- Most common cause of cardiopulmonary arrest in children is *respiratory insufficiency or shock*
- Rhythm disturbances in children are treated only if cardiac output is compromised or the

---

Figure 17–3. Bradycardia decision tree. ABCs, airway, breathing, and circulation; ALS, advanced life support; ET, endotracheal; IO, intraosseous; IV, intravenous. (From American Medical Association: Pediatric Advanced Life Support. JAMA 268(16):2266, 1992. Copyright 1992, American Medical Association.)

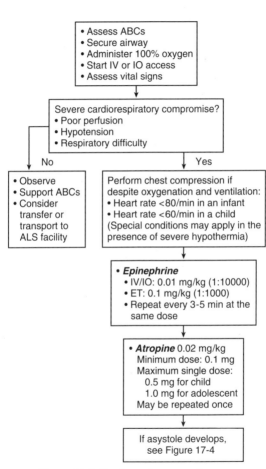

Figure 17-3 *See legend on opposite page*

191

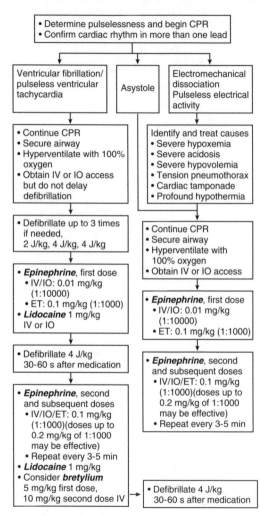

Figure 17-4 *See legend on opposite page*

dysrhythmia has the potential to degenerate to a lethal rhythm.
- Decision trees
  - Pediatric advanced life support
  - Bradycardia (see Fig. 17–3)
  - Asystole and pulseless arrest (see Fig. 17–4)

Bibliography

Barkin R, Rosen P: Emergency Pediatrics: A Guide to Ambulatory Care, 4th ed. St. Louis, Mosby–Year Book, 1994, p. 60.

Chameides L, Hazinski M (eds): Textbook of Pediatric Advanced Life Support. Dallas, TX, American Heart Association, 1994.

Emergency Nurses Association: Emergency Nursing Pediatric Course Instruction Manual. Park Ridge, IL, ENA, 1993.

Emergency Nurses Association: Pediatric Emergency Nursing Resource Guide. Park Ridge, IL, ENA, 1993.

Engel J: Pocket Guide to Pediatric Assessment. St. Louis, CV Mosby, 1989

Ojanen Thomas D: Quick Reference to Pediatric Emergency Nursing. Gaithersburg, MD, Aspen Publishers, Inc., 1991.

Thomas Newman J: Pediatric Nursing, 2nd ed. Springhouse, PA, Springhouse Corporation, 1995.

Figure 17–4. Asystole and pulseless arrest decision tree. CPR, cardiopulmonary resuscitation; ET, endotracheal; IO, intraosseous; IV, intravenous; J, joule. (From American Medical Association: Pediatric Advanced Life Support. JAMA 268(16):266, 1992. Copyright 1992, American Medical Association.)

Chapter 18

Common Emergency Department Procedures

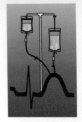

- Procedures vary among institutions. It is expected that the emergency department (ED) nurse is familiar with the equipment and supplies of the particular facility. Refer also to manufacturer's guidelines.
- The following procedures are an overview and may not be all inclusive.

ARTERIAL CANNULATION AND ARTERIAL LINE INSERTION

Indications

- Arterial pressure monitoring
- Repeated arterial blood sampling

Nursing Role

- Radial artery is the most common site
- Assist with positioning
  - Dorsiflex the wrist
- Prepare continuous arterial pressure monitor:

- Prime the tubing with heparinized solution (in IV bag)
- Pressure bag to heparinized IV solution bag
- Calibrate (zero) the monitoring equipment
- Secure arterial cannula with dressing after insertion
- Connect and secure the arterial cannula to pressure monitor tubing
- Secure the wrist to an armboard after procedure
- Ascertain correlation of displayed arterial pressures with manual BP and expected waveforms

Observations

- Arterial pressure waveform display
- Absence of leaking blood at the site or from arterial line
- Hematoma formation at the site
- Circulation, sensation, and movement distal to cannula placement
- Development of complications:
  - Retrograde arterial embolism from rapid retrograde flushing of cannula with more than 3 cc bolus
  - Observe for signs and symptoms of cerebral embolus

ARTERIAL PUNCTURE

Indications

- Obtain heparinized blood for arterial blood gas (ABG) analysis
  - Assesses serum acid-base status
  - Assesses ventilation

- Obtain nonheparinized blood for standard laboratory analysis

Nursing Role/Monitoring

- Use a 20–23 gauge needle for children and adults
- Use a 25 gauge needle for neonates and infants
- Radial artery is preferred site (brachial and femoral sites are also common)
- Identify and localize the site prior to puncture
- Cleanse and prep the area
- Withdraw 1–3 cc of heparinized blood (many ABG kits contain self-filling syringes)
- Apply pressure to the site for at least 5 minutes
- Place specimen on ice and send for processing
- Refer to ABG analysis in Chapter 20

Observations

- Hematoma at the site
- Limited movement, sensation, circulation distal to the puncture site

ARTHROCENTESIS (JOINT ASPIRATION)

Indications

- Swelling or pain in a joint
- Determine cause

Nursing Role/Monitoring

- Aseptic technique is essential
- Prep the skin; shave as indicated
- Provide a new bottle of local anesthetic agent
- Apply dressing to the area

• Administer analgesic agents as ordered

Common aspirated joints

• Knee: position patient on back with the knee extended
• Ankle: position patient on back with foot in a neutral position
• Elbow: position patient with the elbow at a 90° angle. Patient may be supine or prone.

Fluid Analysis

• Cell count
• Gram stain and culture
• Glucose and protein
• Examination for crystals
• Mucin clot (a mixture of glycoproteins that form mucus)

Observations

• Color, movement, and sensation distal to the aspiration site
• Leakage of fluid from the site
• Development of complications
  • Bleeding in the joint
  • Infection

AUTOTRANSFUSION

Indications

• Massive hemothorax
• Transfuses patients with their own shed blood

Contraindications

- Thoracic blood contaminated with bowel contents or infectious materials
- Blood potentially contaminated with malignant cells
- Injury more than 4–6 hours old
- Anticipated autotransfusion of more than 50% of the estimated blood loss

Nursing Role/Monitoring

- Cardiac monitoring
- Pulse oximetry
- Supplemental oxygen
- Follow manufacturer's instructions for type of autotransfusion device used
- Instillation of anticoagulant (i.e., citrate/phosphate/dextrose [CPD]) may be prescribed
  - 1 cc of CPD: 7–10 cc of shed blood
  - Common practice is 60–70 cc of CPD during collection of 500 cc of shed blood
- Monitor time and amount of blood collected and amount of blood reinfused
- Prepare patient for surgical interventions as indicated
- Continuously monitor
  - Fluctuation of fluid
  - Output from chest tube
  - Color of drainage
  - For air leaks (dependent upon closed drainage system used)
- Air leaks can occur
  - From chest drainage system
  - Continued air leak in the lung
  - Esophageal or bronchial injury
  - Incorrectly positioned chest tube

- Tape all tube connections
- Clamping of chest tube during transport not necessary. A tension pneumothorax may develop if the chest tube is clamped before re-expansion of the lung.

Observations

- Signs and symptoms of continued blood loss (shock)
- Subcutaneous emphysema
- Occlusion of chest drainage tubing from
  - Kinks
  - Clots

CENTRAL LINE INSERTION

Indications

- Access to the central veins for
  - Rapid infusion of large amounts of fluid
  - Venous blood sampling
  - Medication administration
  - Obtainment of central venous pressure
- *May be inserted in the ED, or patient may present with these in place*

Types of Central Lines

- Single-, double-, triple-lumen catheters: emergency or short-term central venous (CV) access
- Groshong catheter: long-term CV access
- Hickman catheter
  - Long-term CV access
  - Good for home therapy
- Broviac catheter

- Long-term CV access
- Good for pediatric and elderly patients with small veins
- Hickman/Broviac catheter
  - Long-term CV access
  - Multiple lumens for multiple infusions
- Peripherally inserted central catheter (PICC line)
  - Long-term CV access
  - Good for home therapy
- Implanted ports (see Implanted Vascular Access Device section)

Nursing Role/Monitoring

- Prime the tubing prior to insertion
- Prep the site using strict aseptic technique
- Initiate the IV infusion at keep vein open rate until placement is confirmed by x-ray
- Catheters will be sutured to the skin
- Apply a dressing (a transparent semipermeable membrane is most common)
- PICC lines will need an injection cap for intermittent infusions
- Refer to institutional policy or procedure for accessing existing central lines

Observations

- Chest pain
- Respiratory complaints
  - Dyspnea
  - Respiratory distress
- Signs and symptoms of pneumothorax/hemothorax/pleural effusion
- Signs and symptoms of air embolism
- Thrombosis

- Local infection
- Sepsis

CHEST TUBE INSERTION (CLOSED THORACOSTOMY)

Indications

- Hemothorax
- Pneumothorax
- Tension pneumothorax
- Empyema (generally nonemergent)
- Prophylactic placement in chest trauma patients who require positive pressure ventilation

Nursing Role/Monitoring

- Cardiac monitoring
- Pulse oximetry
- Supplemental oxygen
- Analgesia as ordered
- Consider use of autotransfusion collection chamber if massive hemothorax suspected
- Chest tube size dependent upon
  - Age
  - Weight
  - Condition
  - Pneumothorax (air) = smaller size tube
  - Hemothorax (blood or other fluid) = larger size tube
- Continuously monitor
  - Fluctuation
  - Output
  - Color
  - Air leak
- Air leaks can occur from
  - Chest drainage system

- Continued air leak in the lung
- Esophageal or bronchial injury
- Incorrectly positioned chest tube
- Tape all tube connections
- Obtain specimens of chest tube drainage only from the collection port on the system
- Clamping of chest tube during transport not necessary. A tension pneumothorax may develop if the chest tube is clamped before re-expansion of the lung.

Observations

- Excessive bleeding (>200 cc/hr for 2 hrs) can be from
  - Lung
  - Chest wall
  - Intercostal vessels
  - Mammary vessels
- Subcutaneous emphysema
- Occlusion of chest drainage tubing from
  - Kinks
  - Clots

DIAGNOSTIC PERITONEAL LAVAGE

Indications

- Abdominal trauma/blunt or penetrating: Penetrating trauma may be explored in the OR without ED diagnostic peritoneal lavage
- Suspected intra-abdominal bleeding
- Not useful in suspected retroperitoneal bleeding

Nursing Role/Monitoring

- May use "open" or "closed" technique for peritoneal catheter insertion

- Prior to insertion of peritoneal catheter:
  - Decompress bladder with urinary catheter
  - Decompress stomach with gastric tube
- Withdrawal of gross blood from the peritoneal catheter indicates a positive finding
- If no gross blood is initially aspirated
  - Instill 1 L of warmed lactated Ringer's solution or normal saline rapidly through the catheter
  - Allow the lavage fluid to drain by gravity (drainage collection device must be lower than the abdomen)
- Note color of returned peritoneal fluid
- Send specimen to laboratory for analysis (see Chapter 9)

Observations

- Free flow of fluid by gravity
- Dislodgement of peritoneal catheter

INTRACRANIAL PRESSURE-MONITORING DEVICES

Indications

- Severe head injury
- Risk for complications

Types of Intracranial Pressure (ICP) Monitors

- Intraventricular catheter
- Subarachnoid screw or bolt
- Epidural pressure sensor
- Intradural monitor

Nursing Role/Monitoring

- Cardiac monitoring
- Pulse oximetry
- Supplemental oxygen
- Calibration of ICP monitor according to manufacturer's instructions
- Maintain a normotensive state, influenced by
  - Position
  - Activity
  - Fluids
  - Medications
- Control hemorrhage
- Rapid treatment for increased ICP (refer to Chapter 14)

Observations

- Signs and symptoms of increased ICP
  - Increasing headache
  - Increasing restlessness and decreasing level of consciousness
  - Change in vital signs
  - Eye or pupillary changes
  - Worsening of focal neurologic symptoms
  - New onset of hemiplegia, hemiparesis, or hemianesthesia
- Secure connections between the catheter, stopcocks, transducer, and drainage bag (if present)

IMPLANTED VASCULAR ACCESS DEVICE (VAD)

Indications

- Intermittent infusions
- Long-term IV access for

- IV therapy
- Chemotherapy
- Medication
- Blood products
- Blood sampling
- Not typically used for total parenteral nutrition (TPN) or antibiotics

Nursing Role/Monitoring

- Use only noncore needles with a VAD
  - Right-angle noncoring needle is very common
  - 19 gauge for blood infusion or withdrawal
  - 20 gauge for most other infusions
- Prepare the site prior to access and observe strict aseptic technique
- Palpate the area to locate the VAD
- Insert the needle at the center of the device perpendicular to the port (if top access device) or parallel (if side-entry access device); push through the skin and port until the needle touches bottom of the VAD reservoir
- Aspirate for blood return

Observations

- Inability to flush the VAD
  - Kinked tubing
  - Closed clamp
  - Kinked catheter
- Site infection
- Skin breakdown
- Extravasation of injected fluid
- Thrombosis

LUMBAR PUNCTURE (LP)

Indications

- Rule out central nervous system infection
- Potential increased ICP is ruled out prior to performance of LP
- If any question of increased ICP, a computed tomography (CT) scan is obtained prior to LP

Nursing Role/Monitoring

- Proper positioning of the patient is crucial
  - Patient is placed near the edge of stretcher
  - Maintain in a position with neck flexed and knees drawn upward (fetal position)
  - Place one arm behind the patient's knees and the other behind the patient's neck
  - Shoulders and back are perpendicular to the stretcher
  - An alternative position is to have the patient sitting, dangle legs over the side of the stretcher, bending over forward at the waist with the neck flexed; face the patient and hold in this position
- Children less than 5 years old will require a 22 gauge, 1½-inch needle
Instruct older children and adults to lie flat after the procedure
Label cerebrospinal fluid (CSF) tubes as directed or as follows:
  - Tube #1 = culture and Gram stain
  - Tube #2 = protein and glucose
  - Tube #3 = cell count
  - Tube #4 = miscellaneous tests
- Refer to Chapter 9 for interpretation of results

Observations

- Development of respiratory distress or cardiorespiratory arrest, which may result from holding the patient (especially children) too tightly
- Development of postprocedure headache (rare in small children and infants)
- Leakage of CSF or blood from the puncture site

NASAL PACKING

Indications

- Control of epistaxis
- Usually used if direct pressure and cautery have been unsuccessful

Nursing Role/Monitoring

- Instruct the patient to blow nose or suction nares
- Application of cold packs to nose or neck is generally ineffective
- Ensure adequate lighting
- Obtain nasal speculum
- Monitor patient's heart rate and blood pressure during the procedure
- Consider the use of a cardiac monitor for high-risk patients when using cocaine, lidocaine, epinephrine, or phenylephrine solutions for local anesthesia (example: elderly and known cardiac patients)

Anterior Nasal Packing

- 72 inches of ¼ to ½ inch petrolatum-impregnated gauze.
  - Other nostril may be packed to prevent displacement of the nasal septum

- Commercial products such as nasal tampons or hemostatic nasal balloons may be used.
  - Provide antibiotic ointment to decrease risk of infection

OBSERVATIONS

- Signs of infection at 24, 48, and 72-hour follow-up appointments
- Compliance with antibiotic regime until packing is removed
- Understanding of discharge instructions after observing the patient for 30 minutes after packing

Posterior Nasal Packing

- Gauze packs may be inserted through the mouth and pulled up tightly into the nasopharynx with a string
- 16-gauge foley catheters with 5 or 30 cc balloons are inflated with air in the nasopharynx
- Anterior packings can be placed against the posterior packs
- Commercial preparations are available

NURSING ROLE/MONITORING

- Keep a 20–30 cc syringe taped to the stretcher for immediate balloon deflation
- Administer humidified oxygen
- Monitor vital signs
- Record amount of blood loss
- Monitor hemoglobin and hematocrit
- Obtain platelet and coagulation studies
- Prepare for admission

OBSERVATIONS

- Airway obstruction
- Hypoventilation
- Hypovolemia due to excessive blood loss

PERICARDIOCENTESIS

Indications

- Removal of fluid in the pericardial sac because of
  - Pericardial effusion
  - Infection
  - Hemorrhage (traumatic pericardial tamponade)
- Procedure may be therapeutic or diagnostic

Nursing Role/Monitoring

- Cardiac monitor
- Pulse oximeter
- Supplemental oxygen
- Continuously monitor vital signs
- Echocardiogram in the stable patient may be used to establish presence of pericardial effusion (ultrasound may also diagnose this finding)
- Pericardiocentesis in the unstable patient is a life-saving procedure, followed by definitive surgical interventions
- Position the patient supine, in reverse Trendelenburg at a 45 degree angle
- Attach the patient to a 12-lead EKG machine
- Attach one end of an alligator clip to a metal spinal needle (3 inch) and the other end of the alligator clip to a V lead of the EKG machine
- Prep and drape the subxiphoid area
- Observe the EKG machine and monitor the V lead during insertion of the needle for

- ST segment elevation (ventricular epicardial contact)
- PR segment elevation (atrial epicardial contact)
- Record the amount of blood aspirated from the pericardial sac (Note: blood will not immediately clot due to defibrinization by mechanical action of the contracting heart)

Observations

- Pneumothorax
- Coronary artery injury or myocardial laceration
- Arrhythmias
- Return of pericardial tamponade
  - Decreased arterial pressure
  - Increased venous pressure
  - Muffled, distant heart sounds

OPEN THORACOTOMY

Indications

- Pulselessness due to trauma
- Permits direct massage of the heart, cross-clamping of the aorta, and other indicated surgical procedures
- Consider potential for meaningful survival

Nursing Role/Monitoring

- ABCs
- Cardiac monitoring
- Pulse oximetry
- Supplemental oxygen
- Assure personal protective equipment (including booties/eye protection) for all involved in the procedure

- Rapid fluid resuscitation (with use of rapid infuser or pressure bags)
- Prepare for possible internal defibrillation (maximum voltage = 50 joules)
- Prepare for possible 30cc balloon catheter insertion (for penetrating cardiac wound)
- Notify the operating room

Observations

- Time the aorta is cross-clamped
- Spontaneous return of mechanical contractions with electrical impulses

Bibliography

American Medical Association: Guidelines for cardiopulmonary resuscitation and emergency cardiac care. JAMA 268:2135–2298, 1992.

Budassi Sheehy S: Manual of Emergency Care. St. Louis, CV Mosby, 1990.

Budassi Sheehy S, Marvin JA, LeDoc Jimmerson C: Manual of Clinical Trauma Care, The First Hour. St. Louis, CV Mosby, 1989.

Burrell ZL, Owens Burrell L: Critical Care. St. Louis, CV Mosby, 1977.

Emergency Nurses Association: Trauma Nursing Core Course Instructor Manual. Park Ridge, IL, ENA 1995.

Kelly W, et al (eds): IV Therapy. Springhouse, PA, Springhouse Corp., 1990.

Kitt S, Selfridge-Thomas J, Proehl J, Kaiser J: Emergency Nursing: A Physiologic and Clinical Perspective, 2nd ed. Philadelphia, WB Saunders, 1995.

Selfridge-Thomas J: Manual of Emergency Nursing. Philadelphia, WB Saunders, 1995.

Vander Salm TJ (ed): Atlas of Bedside Procedures. Boston, Little, Brown, 1979.

Chapter 19

Psychiatric and Psychologic Emergencies

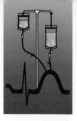

SUICIDE RISK ASSESSMENT FOR THE ED: SAD PERSONS

- S = **S**ex
- A = **A**ge
- D = **D**epression
- P = **P**revious attempts
- E = **E**TOH (ethanol)
- R = **R**ational thinking loss
- S = **S**ocial supports lacking
- O = **O**rganized plan
- N = **N**o spouse
- S = **S**ickness

ASSESSMENT FOR PSYCHIATRIC AND PSYCHOLOGIC ILLNESS

- Assure physiologic stability
- Obtain a history
- Perform physical and mental status examination
  - Behavior and general appearance
  - Speech
  - Mood and affect
  - Thought process and content

- Perception
- Judgment and insight
- Cognitive ability
- Impulse control
- Reliability
- Assess for organic illness that can produce psychiatric symptoms
- Assess for chemical use that can produce psychiatric symptoms

PSYCHIATRIC AND PSYCHOLOGIC PRESENTATIONS

- Anxiety
- Depression (manic or bipolar)
- Psychosis (paranoia, schizophrenia)
- Suicidal ideation or attempt (see SAD PERSONS)
- Violent behavior
- Neurosis
- Dysfunctional grieving

EXTRAPYRAMIDAL REACTIONS

- Dystonias
- Akathisia
- Akinesia
- Side effects of antipsychotic medications

Treatment

- Diphenhydramine hydrochloride (Benadryl) 25–50 mg IM or IV
- Benztropine mesylate (Cogentin) 2 mg IM or IV
- Supportive environment

Substance-Related Reactions

(see Chapter 21)

Bibliography

Holmes T, Rahe R: The social readjustment rating scale. J Psychosom Res 11:213, 1967.

Joint Commission Accreditation of Health Care Organizations: Accreditation Manual for Hospitals. Chicago, JCAHCO, 1995.

Patterson W, Dohn HH, Bird J, et al: Evaluation of suicidal patients: The SAD PERSONS scale. Psychosomatics 24:343, 1983.

Taylor C: Essentials of Psychiatric Nursing. St. Louis, CV Mosby, 1990.

Chapter 20

Respiratory Emergencies

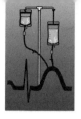

VENTILATION

Breath Sounds (see Table 20–1)

Indications for Mechanical Ventilation

- Pao_2 less than 50 mm Hg with FIO_2 more than 60%
- $Paco_2$ greater than 50 mm Hg with pH less than 7.25

Oxygen Administration Devices
(see Table 20–2)

Types of Ventilators

- Positive-pressure ventilators
  - Inflate lungs by exerting positive pressure on airway
  - Exhalation is passive
- Pressure-cycled ventilators
  - Inspiration ends when a preset pressure is reached
  - Volume of air or oxygen may vary as the patient's airway resistance changes
- Time-cycled ventilators
  - Inspiration ends when a preset time is reached

Table 20–1. Breath Sounds

Type	Location	Associated Problems	Description
Vesicular	In most of lungs peripheral areas	Normal	Low pitch, soft
Bronchial	Over trachea	Normal	Hollow, high pitched, harsh
Bronchovesicular	Main bronchus	Normal	Tubular, medium pitch
Crackles (rales)	Peripheral airways Alveoli	Inflammation, congestion, excess fluid, excess mucus	Fine or coarse crackles or popping sound, usually at end of inspiration, may be both inspiratory and expiratory
Rhonchi	Large airways	Inflammation, excess fluid, excess mucus	Sibilant (musical), sonorous (snoring, wheezing) usually louder with expiration, may clear somewhat with cough
Wheeze	Large or small airways	Bronchoconstriction due to bronchospasm, fluid, mucus, inflammation, lesion	High or low pitch, usually expiratory, may be inspiratory and expiratory

Table 20-2. Oxygen Administration Devices

Device	Oxygen Concentration (%)	Flow Rate (L/min)
Nasal cannula	24–30	1–2
	30–40	3–5
	42–44	6
Simple mask	40–60	8–10
Partial rebreather mask	50–75	8–12
Nonrebreather mask	60–90	12–15
Venturi mask	24, 26, 28	4–6
	30, 35, 40	6–8
Tracheostomy collar	30–100	8–10
T-piece	30–100	8–10
Bag-valve-mask with reservoir	60–100	15

- Volume is regulated by length of inspiration and flow rate
- Used primarily in neonates and infants
- Volume-cycled ventilators
  - Inspiration ends when a preset volume is reached
  - Volume of air and oxygen is consistent despite varying airway pressures
  - Most commonly used ventilator (e.g., MA-1, Bear, Servo)

Modes of Ventilation

- Controlled: ventilator completely controls patient's ventilation according to TV and RR
- Assist/control: patient triggers ventilator; if patient does not take a breath, ventilator delivers a breath at minimum rate and volume
- Intermittent mandatory ventilation (IMV): patient breathes spontaneously while ventilator provides preset FIO_2 and additional breaths to ensure adequate ventilation

Problems with Ventilators
(see Table 20–3)

Continous Positive Airway Pressure (CPAP)

- For patients breathing spontaneously, CPAP
  - Can adequately ventilate, but cannot effectively oxygenate because of decreased functional reserve capacity (FRC)
  - Can help patients with secretions blocking the airway or with fluid-filled alveoli
  - Also used to treat refractory hypoxemia resulting from atelectasis
- A tight-fitting, continous flow face mask is necessary
- Careful assessment of cardiovascular and ventilatory status during CPAP is necessary
- Consider insertion of NG tube to decrease risk of gastric dilatation, vomiting, and aspiration
- Usually tolerated for 12–36 hours

Table 20–3. Troubleshooting Ventilators

Problem	Intervention
Pressure alarm	Assess for plugged/occluded tube
	Suction airway for secretions
	Empty condensation fluid
	Assess for kinked tubing
	Reposition the patient
	Insert oral airway
	Assess for hypoxia or bronchospasm
	Adjust sensitivity
	Assess patient's need for sedation
Volume alarm	Assess for leak in ET tube cuff
	Assess for leak or disconnection in ventilator tubing

MNEMONIC FOR TREATMENT OF PULMONARY EDEMA: MOST DAMP

- M = **M**orphine
- O = **O**xygen
- S = **S**itting upright position
- T = **T**ourniquets (rotating tourniquets no longer used, a "chemical tourniquet" is likened to the use of nitroglycerin)
- D = **D**iuretics
- A = **A**minophylline
- M = **M**onitor
- P = **P**ositive pressure ventilation

Pulse Oximetry

- Measures percentage of hemoglobin saturated with oxygen (SpO_2)
- Normal = 98%
- Saturation of hemoglobin is calculated by the pulse oximeter based on the differential absorption of light by the patient's oxyhemoglobin
- Factors affecting SpO_2 measurements:
  - Decreased perfusion
  - Hypothermia
  - Incorrect placement of probe or sensor
  - Vasoconstriction
  - Movement of patient (tremors, seizures)
  - Lighting fluctuations
  - Methemoglobin, carboxyhemoglobin

SpO_2 and PO_2 (see Table 20–4)

VENTILATION-PERFUSION (V̇/Q̇) MATCHES

- Normal ventilation matches perfusion
  - Healthy lung
  - A given amount of blood bypasses an alveolus and is matched with an equal amount of gas
  - Ratio = 1:1
- Low ventilation-perfusion ratio
  - Shunt-producing disorders
  - Perfusion exceeds ventilation
  - Blood bypasses alveoli without gas exchange
  - Seen with obstruction of distal airways
    - Pneumonia
    - Atelectasis
    - Tumor
    - Mucus plug

Table 20–4. Correlation Between SpO$_2$ and Po$_2$

Po$_2$	SpO$_2$
100	97
90	97
80	96
70	94
60	91
50	85
40	74
30	57

Based on the oxyhemoglobin dissociation curve, the SpO$_2$ may be correlated to the Po$_2$ (assuming temperature = 37.0°C, Paco$_2$ = 40, pH = 7.40, normal levels of 2,3, DPG, and adult hemoglobin).

- High ventilation-perfusion ratio
  - Dead space–producing disorders
  - Ventilation exceeds perfusion
  - Dead space occurs
  - Alveoli have inadequate blood supply to allow gas exchange
  - Seen with
    - Pulmonary emboli
    - Pulmonary infarction
    - Cardiogenic shock
- Silent unit
  - Absence of (or limited) ventilation and perfusion
  - Seen with
    - Pneumothorax
    - Acute respiratory distress syndrome (ARDS)
- Arterial-Alveolar (a-A) ratio shunt calculation:

$$\text{a-A ratio} = \frac{PaO_2}{PAO_2}$$

PNEUMOTHORAX (OPEN/SUCKING)

- Air enters the pleural space
- Surgical or traumatic wound
- Atmospheric air is sucked into the pleural cavity
- Lung collapses on the affected side as negative pressure becomes more positive

PNEUMOTHORAX (CLOSED)

- Air enters the pleural space through the lung (i.e., ruptured bleb)
- Pleural pressure increases
- Lung expansion is prevented

HEMOTHORAX

- Results from penetrating or blunt trauma
- Rupture of large vessels can result in massive blood loss
- Blood collects in the pleural space

TENSION PNEUMOTHORAX

- A result of continued, unrelieved intrapleural pressure
- Affected lung collapses and shifts toward the mediastinum
- May result in compression of the great vessels and heart if not treated stat

MANAGEMENT OF PNEUMOTHORAX

Signs and Symptoms of Pneumothorax

- Dyspnea or shortness of breath
- Chest pain

- History of trauma (or may be atraumatic, i.e., spontaneous)
- May exhibit symptoms of shock
  - Hypotension
  - Tachycardia
- Diminished lung sounds on affected side
- Evidence on x-ray of pneumothorax, tension pneumothorax, hemothorax
- May have mediastinal shift

Treatment of Pneumothorax

- ABCs
- High-flow oxygen
- Chest tube insertion (see Chapter 18)
- Cardiac monitor
- Pulse oximeter
- IV fluids

ASTHMA

- Obstructive pulmonary disease
- Bronchial inflammation and smooth muscle contraction are significant characteristics
- Also characterized by
  - Airway hyperactivity
  - Reversible bronchospasm
  - Mucosal edema
  - Excessive mucus production
- Degree of obstruction determines severity of symptoms
- Patients with increased risk
  - Prior intensive care admissions
  - Prior intubations
  - Maintenance steroid therapy
  - Lung disease

Assessment

- Dyspnea
  - Use of accessory muscles
  - Nasal flaring
  - Retractions
  - Wheezing (expiratory or inspiratory)
  - Air entry/exchange
  - Peak expiratory flow rate (PEFR)
  - Cough (dry or productive)
- Hypoxia
  - Restlessness, fatigue
  - Pulsus paradoxus
  - Tachypnea
  - Tachycardia
  - Pallor, cyanosis
  - Diaphoresis
- History
  - Previous asthma treatment, admissions, at-home management, and episodic care
  - Presence of high-risk factors (see high risks previously)
  - Antecedent illness
  - Allergies
  - Length of current wheezing episode
- Measurement of bronchospasm
  - FEV_1: spirometry to determine forced end-expiratory volume in one second
  - PEFR: increased probability for admission exists when PEFR is less than 20% predicted *before* treatment and less than 60% predicted *after* treatment (see Fig. 20–1)

Asthma Management in the ED

- Beta-agonist therapy
  - Aerosolized via nebulizer

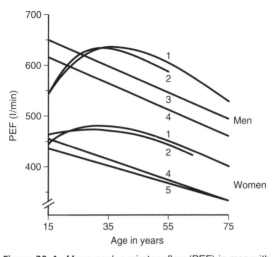

Figure 20–1. Mean peak expiratory flow (PEF) in men with height of 175 cm and women with height of 160 cm derived from new regression equations and compared with those described by others. For men, 1 = present series; 2 = Gregg and Nunn 1973; 3 = Leiner et al.; 4 = European Community for Coal and Steel. For women, 1 = present series; 2 = Gregg and Nunn 1973; 3 = Leiner et al.; 4 = European Community for Coal and Steel; 5 = Peltzer and Thomson. (From Nunn AJ, Gregg I: New regression equation for predicting peak expiratory flow in adults. Brit Med J 298:1067, 1989.)

- Major agents are albuterol and metaproterenol
- Side effect of tachycardia may limit back-to-back or continous administration
- Steroids
  - Inhibit inflammatory component
  - Used *early* in treatment

225

- Methylprednisolone 2 mg/kg/dose IV initially; 0.5–1.0 mg/kg/dose q6h IV, given IV push over one to several minutes
- Chest x-ray: only when pneumonia, foreign body, pneumothorax suspected
- Antibiotics only when bacterial infection identified
- Indications for intubation
  - Exhaustion
  - Worsening hypoxia despite agressive ED treatment
- ED therapies to consider:
  - Epinephrine
  - Magnesium
  - Helium/oxygen mixtures
  - Inhaled anesthetics
  - Theophylline infusions
  - Terbutaline infusions
  - Anticholinergics
    - Atropine
    - Ipratropium

ARTERIAL BLOOD GAS (ABG) STUDIES

- Measures blood pH, arterial oxygen tension (Pao_2), and carbon dioxide tension ($Paco_2$)
- Pao_2 indicates oxygenation of blood
- $Paco_2$ indicates adequacy of alveolar ventilation
- Useful in determining the ability of kidneys to reabsorb or excrete bicarbonate ions (HCO_3) to maintain a normal pH

Interpretation of ABG Values
(see Table 20–5)

- Step one: What is the pH?
  - Determine if the pH is increased or decreased

Table 20-5. Normal Values

	Arterial	Capillary	Venous
pH	7.35–7.45	7.35–7.45	7.31–7.41
PaO_2	80–100	40–60	35–40
$PaCO_2$	35–45	35–45	41–51
HCO_3	22–26	22–26	22–26
BE	± 2	± 2	± 2
Acid/Base	pH 7.35–7.45	Increased pH = alkalosis >7.45 Decreased pH = acidosis <7.35	
Metabolic component	Bicarbonate HCO_3 22–26 mEq	Increased HCO_3 = metabolic alkalosis >26 mEq Decreased HCO_3 = metabolic acidosis <22 mEq	
Respiratory component	$PaCO_2$ 35–40 mm Hg	Increased $PaCO_2$ = respiratory acidosis >40 mm Hg Decreased $PaCO_2$ = respiratory alkalosis <35 mm Hg	

- Increase indicates alkalosis; decrease indicates acidosis.
- Step two: What is the primary cause of the acid-base disturbance?
  - Match the abnormal pH with the abnormal component
    - Respiratory: $Paco_2$
    - Metabolic: HCO_3
  - Example
    - pH = 7.50: alkalosis
    - $Paco_2$ = 25: alkalosis
    - HCO_3 = 24: normal
  - The above example is respiratory alkalosis. The respiratory component is deranged in the same manner as the pH (alkalosis).
  - Most ABGs will not be this obvious. The body compensates to correct abnormal acid-base conditions.
- Step three: Has compensation occurred?
  - Determine if the ABG demonstrates a compensated, uncompensated, or partially compensated acid-base balance
  - Example
    - pH = 7.32: acidosis
    - $Paco_2$ = 30: respiratory alkalosis
    - HCO_3 = 16: metabolic acidosis
  - The pH reflects an acidosis
  - The pH and HCO_3 match, thus step two tells us the patient has metabolic acidosis.
  - The respiratory component is deranged in the opposite manner (alkalosis), which tells us the body is attempting to compensate for the metabolic acidosis.
  - The body has not completely compensated. In the presence of complete compensation, the pH would be within normal limits (near 7.40); thus

there is a partially compensated metabolic acidosis.
- Step four: Is oxygenation adequate?
  - Determine if the PaO_2 is within normal limits
  - If less than 80 torr, hypoxemia also exists

Examples

- Respiratory alkalosis (uncompensated)
  - pH ↑
  - $PaCO_2$ ↓
  - HCO_3 normal
- Respiratory alkalosis (partially compensated)
  - pH ↑
  - $PaCO_2$ ↓
  - HCO_3 ↓
- Metabolic alkalosis (uncompensated)
  - pH ↑
  - $PaCO_2$ normal
  - HCO_3 ↑
- Metabolic alkalosis (partially compensated)
  - pH ↑
  - $PaCO_2$ ↑
  - HCO_3 ↑
- Respiratory acidosis (uncompensated)
  - pH ↓
  - $PaCO_2$ ↑
  - HCO_3 normal
- Respiratory acidosis (partially compensated)
  - pH ↓
  - $PaCO_2$ ↑
  - HCO_3 ↓
- Metabolic acidosis (uncompensated)
  - pH ↓
  - $PaCO_2$ normal
  - HCO_3 ↓

- Metabolic acidosis (partially compensated)
  - pH ↓
  - $Paco_2$ ↓
  - HCO_3 ↓
- Combined respiratory and metabolic acidosis
  - pH ↓
  - $Paco_2$ ↑
  - HCO_3 ↓
- Combined respiratory and metabolic alkalosis
  - pH ↑
  - $Paco_2$ ↓
  - HCO_3 ↑

EFFECTS OF OXYGEN ADMINISTRATION

- Elevates alveolar and arterial oxygen tension
- Hemoglobin saturation increases
- Arterial oxygen content increases
- Results in improved tissue oxygenation

Duration of "E" Tanks
(see Table 20–6)

Table 20–6. Duration of "E" Tanks at Various Flow Rates (Full Tank)

Rate (L/min)	Will Last (hrs)
2	5.1
3	3.4
4	2.5
5	2.0
6	1.7
7	1.4

Bibliography

Budassi Sheehy S: Emergency Nursing Principles and Practice, 3rd ed. St. Louis, Mosby–Year Book, 1992.

Kitt S, Selfridge-Thomas J, Proehl J, Kaiser J: Emergency Nursing: A Physiologic and Clinical Perspective. Philadelphia, WB Saunders, 1995.

Loeb S (ed): Respiratory Support. Springhouse, PA, Springhouse Corp., 1991.

Markovchick V, Pons P: Emergency Medicine Secrets. Philadelphia, Hanley & Belfus, Inc., 1993.

Selfridge-Thomas J: Manual of Emergency Nursing. Philadelphia, WB Saunders, 1995.

Smeltzer S, Bare B: Brunner and Suddarth's Textbook of Medical Surgical Nursing. Philadelphia, JB Lippincott, 1992.

Task Force on Interhospital Transport: Guidelines for Air and Ground Transport of Neonatal and Pediatric Patients. Elk Grove Village, American Academy of Pediatrics, 1993.

Chapter 21
Substance Abuse

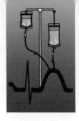

ETHANOL

- Most commonly used intoxicant
- Depresses the CNS
- Augments gamma-aminobutyric acid (GABA) mediated synaptic inhibition
- Chronic drinkers develop tolerance to alcohol and may have higher levels before exhibiting signs or symptoms of intoxication.
- Alcohol metabolizes at approximately 25 mg/dL/hr

Blood Alcohol Levels (BAL)

- 25 mg/dL: impaired judgment
- 50 mg/dL: affects gross motor control and orientation
- 100 mg/dL: considered "intoxicated"

Clinical Effects of Alcohol Use

- Flushing of skin
- Tachycardia
- Increased sweating
- Mydriasis
- Dysarthria
- Incoordination
- Change in level of consciousness
- Emotional lability

- Impaired cardiac output
- Arrhythmias
- Nausea and vomiting
- Coma
- Death

Systemic Effects of Alcoholism

- Chronic drinking affects
  - Eyes
  - GI system
  - GU system
  - Endocrine and metabolic functions
  - Neurologic functions
  - Cardiovascular systems
- May contribute to
  - Cancers
  - Psychiatric disorders
  - Hematologic disorders

Alcoholic Ketoacidosis (AKA)

- Typical presentation to the ED
  - Chronic drinker
  - Recent heavy drinking
  - Cuts down on alcohol and food due to GI complaints
  - Suffers a loss of carbohydrates and depleted glycogen stores

PATHOPHYSIOLOGIC EFFECTS OF AKA

- Body mobilizes fat from adipose tissue
- There is a mediated response of a decrease in insulin and an increase in glucagon, catecholamines, growth hormones, and cortisol
- Fatty acids are oxidized

233

- Acetyl coenzyme A is converted to acetoacetate
- Acetoacetate is converted to beta-hydroxybutyrate in AKA

PATHOPHYSIOLOGIC CAUSES OF AKA

- Volume depletion that interferes with renal elimination of acetoacetate and beta-hydroxybutyrate
- May have lactic acidosis due to hypoperfusion
- pH may be normal due to compensatory respiratory alkalosis or primary metabolic alkalosis due to vomiting
- Assay for ketones in the patient with AKA may be only mildly positive

TREATMENT FOR AKA

- Fluid replacement
- Glucose
- Thiamine

Alcohol Withdrawal
(see Table 21–1)

- Withdrawal from alcohol is a potentially lethal process.
- Mortality rate for withdrawal is 5–15%
- Symptoms begin approximately eight hours after the last drink
- Induction of withdrawal symptoms in an individual with significant BAL can occur by dropping that BAL by 25% at a rapid rate (e.g., BAL of 300 rapidly dropped to 225 may induce withdrawal symptoms).
- A rapid drop in BAL may occur after rapid IV infusions

Table 21–1. Stages of Alcohol Withdrawal

Stage	Signs and Symptoms
I	Tremors
	Tachycardia
	Hypertension
	Perspiration
	Anorexia
	Insomnia
	Hyperthermia
II	Intensification of Stage I symptoms
	Hallucinations (auditory, visual, kinesthetic)
III	Stage I & II symptoms
	Delusions
	Disorientation
	Delirium
	Amnesia
IV	Seizure activity

Modified with permission from Cook L: Substance abuse emergencies. *In* Emergency Nurses Association: Emergency Nursing Core Curriculum, 4th ed. Philadelphia, WB Saunders, 1994.

Alcohol Screening
(see Table 21–2)

COCAINE

- Smoked (crack, freebase)
- Snorted
- Used intravenously

Common Street Names for Cocaine

- Coke
- Crack

Table 21-2. The Brief Michigan Alcoholism Screening Test

Question	Circle correct answer		Points
1. Do you feel you are a normal drinker?	Yes	No	N2
2. Do friends or relatives think you are a normal drinker?	Yes	No	N2
3. Have you ever attended a meeting of Alcoholics Anonymous?	Yes	No	Y5
4. Have you ever lost friends or girlfriends/boyfriends because of drinking?	Yes	No	Y2
5. Have you ever gotten into trouble at work because of drinking?	Yes	No	Y2
6. Have you ever neglected your obligations, your family, or your work for 2 or more days in a row because you were drinking?	Yes	No	Y2

7. Have you ever had delirium tremens (DTs) or severe shaking, or heard voices or seen things that weren't there after heavy drinking?	Yes	No	Y2
8. Have you ever gone to anyone for help about your drinking?	Yes	No	Y5
9. Have you ever been in a hospital because of drinking?	Yes	No	Y5
10. Have you ever been arrested for drunk driving or driving after drinking?	Yes	No	Y2
Score 6 = probable diagnosis of alcoholism			

From Pokorny AL, Miller BA, Kaplan HB: The brief MAST: A shortened version of the Michigan Alcoholism Screening Test. Am J Psychiatry 129:342–345, 1972. Copyright 1972, American Psychiatric Association; with permission.

- Speedball (mixed with heroin)
- Paste/pasta/bazooka
- Snow

Clinical Effects of Cocaine

CARDIAC EFFECTS

- Tachycardia
- Bradycardia
- Arrhythmias
- Angina
- Myocardial infarction (MI)
- Endocarditis

RESPIRATORY EFFECTS

- Bronchitis
- Pneumonia
- Pneumothorax
- Pulmonary edema

VENOUS EFFECTS

- Vasculitis
- Deep vein thrombosis (DVT)

METABOLIC EFFECTS

- Weight loss
- Hyperthermia

NOSE AND THROAT EFFECTS

- Epistaxis
- Ulcerations
- Septal perforations
- Sinusitis

GASTROINTESTINAL EFFECTS

- Nausea
- Vomiting
- Abdominal pain
- Bleeding
- Pancreatitis
- Cirrhosis

SKIN EFFECTS

- Coke burns
- Phlebitis

EMERGENCY TREATMENT FOR COCAINE ABUSE

- ABCs
- Treat the symptoms
- EKG
- Sedation if severely agitated

Lysergic Acid Diethylamide (LSD)

- A psychedelic/hallucinogen
  - Causes subjective distortions of reality
  - Results in perception of things that do not really exist
  - Hallucinations may be
    - Visual
    - Auditory
    - Tactile
    - Olfactory

CLINICAL EFFECTS OF LSD

- Agitation
- Dysphoria

- Hypertension
- Tachycardia
- Hyperthermia

- ABCs
- IV fluids with dextrose and thiamine
- Consider naloxone if respiratory depression
- Quiet location with minimal stimuli
- Gentle reorientation
- Sedation if needed

Marijuana

STREET NAMES FOR MARIJUANA

- Grass
- Mary Jane (MJ)
- Joint; stick
- Hemp
- Cannabis
- Reefer
- Weed
- Wacky weed
- Hashish/hash/kif (dried resin that is smoked)
- Pot
- Bhang

CLINICAL EFFFECTS OF MARIJUANA

- Psychiatric effects
  - Euphoria, elation, relaxation, dreaminess, feeling of well-being, laughing, silliness
  - Altered thought processes, impaired judgment
  - Increased awareness of stimuli
  - Altered concepts of time, space, body image

- Speech changes
- Physical effects
  - Chest tightness
  - Head pressure
  - Increased appetite and thirst
  - Ataxia
  - Tremor
  - Tachycardia
- Marijuana may remain detectable in the urine an average of 27 days or longer after cessation

EMERGENCY TREATMENT FOR MARIJUANA ABUSE

- ABCs
- Treat the symptoms
- Supportive, nonjudgmental environment

OPOIDS (see Table 21–3)

STREET NAMES FOR HEROIN

- Dope
- Skag

Table 21–3. Types of Opioid Substances

Natural	Semisynthetic	Synthetic
Morphine	Heroin	Meperidine
Codeine	Hydromorphone	Methadone
	Oxymorphone	Levorphanol tartrate
	Oxycodone	Paregoric
		Diphenoxylate
		Fentanyl
		Propoxyphene

- Shill
- Horse
- "H"
- White stuff
- Lady Jane

TERMS RELATED TO OPIOID USE

- Jones: opioid withdrawal
- Junkie: addict
- Mainlining: IV injection
- Skin popping: intradermal injection
- Works: syringe equipment
- Chipping: occasional use

CLINICAL EFFECTS OF OPIOID USE

- Respiratory depression
- CNS depression
- Hypotension
- Bradycardia

TREATMENT FOR OPIOID ABUSE

- ABCs
- Naloxone 2 mg IV push up to 10–20 mg if severe opioid overdose

Bibliography

Emergency Nurses Association: Emergency Nursing Core Curriculum, 4th ed. Philadelphia, WB Saunders, 1994.

Goldfrank L, Flomenbaum N, Lewin N, et al: Goldfrank's Toxicologic Emergencies, 5th ed. Norwalk, Appleton & Lange, 1994.

Pokorny AL, Miller BA, Kaplan HB: The brief MAST: A shortened version of the Michigan Alcoholism Screening Test. Am J Psychiatry 129:342–345, 1972.

Chapter 22
Surface Traumas

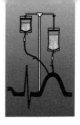

TREATMENT FOR SURFACE TRAUMA

- Assess color, movement, sensation, and pulses distal to the wound
- Consider local anesthesia if needed for thorough cleansing (see Chapter 11)
- Cleanse thoroughly, and, if necessary, debride to prevent tattooing of skin
- Obtain hemostasis as indicated, with direct or indirect pressure
- Elevate affected areas
- Close wound as indicated
- Apply sterile dressings (range from adhesive bandage to bulky dressings)
- Give antibiotics as indicated
- Instruct for wound recheck, home care, and suture removal
- Tetanus prophylaxis

BITES

Human Bites

- Considered a "dirty" wound
  - Multiple organisms in mouth, saliva, and on teeth

243

- Closure is dependent upon severity of the wound due to high risk for infection
- May have teeth marks, ecchymosis, swelling
- May require IV antibiotics if severe

Animal Bites

- Reportable to local police or animal control
- Canine teeth can cause deep puncture wounds or tear skin
  - Closure is dependent upon severity of the wound
  - High risk for infection
- Rabies can be carried by
  - Raccoons
  - Bats
  - Squirrels
  - Skunks
  - Opossums
  - Cats
  - Dogs

Rabies Postexposure Treatment

RABIES IMMUNE GLOBULIN (RIG), HUMAN (HYPERAB, IMOGAM)

- Dosage for adults and children:
  - 20 units/kg IM
    - Infiltrate one-half the dose locally around the wound
    - Give the remainder IM (gluteal)
- Given with Human Diploid Cell Cultures Rabies Vaccine (HDCV)

RABIES VIRUS VACCINE, HUMAN DIPLOID CELL VACCINE (HDCV) (IMOVAX)

- Dosage: 1 mL IM on days 0, 3, 7, 14, and 28
  - Given IM only

Snake Bites

Know the snakes in your geographic area.

TYPES OF SNAKE

- Pit viper
  - Rattlesnake
  - Cottonmouth
  - Copperhead
  - Water moccasin
- Elapids
  - Coral snake
  - Cobra
- Viperids: puff adder
- Hydrophids: sea snakes
- Colubrids: boomslang
- How to tell a coral snake (poisonous) from similar looking nonpoisonous snakes

    Red touch yellow

    Kill a fellow

    Red touch black

    Okay for Jack

- Colors refer to the bands on the snake

VENOMS

- Cause tissue destruction
- Injected via snake fangs (manufactured in salivary glands, stored in the fangs)

- Some venoms are cardiotoxic, neurotoxic, hemotoxic, or combination of two

NATIONAL ANTIVENIN INDEX:
(405) 271-5454

Arachnid and Insect Bites and Stings

BLACK WIDOW SPIDERS

- Black body
- Red hourglass on abdomen
- Neurotoxic venom
- Treat the symptoms, which may include shock

BROWN RECLUSE SPIDERS

- Light brown body
- Dark brown fiddle shape on back
- Local reactions:
  - Edema
  - Bluish ring around the bite area
  - Bleb formation
- Systemic reactions:
  - Fever
  - Nausea or vomiting
  - Weakness
  - Joint pain
  - Petechiae
  - Severe signs of shock, disseminated intravascular coagulation (DIC), cardiac arrest
- Treat the symptoms
- Support ABCs
- Patient may need blood transfusions

BEES (BUMBLE, HONEY), WASPS, HORNETS, FIRE ANTS

- Remove the stinger (if any)
  - Scrape with a credit card or stiff cardboard
  - Do not use forceps to grasp (may inject more venom)
- Treat local reactions with
  - Ice bag
  - Elevation
  - Antihistamines
- More severe reactions (anaphylaxis) may require following treatment:
  - ABCs
  - Epinephrine
  - Vasopressors
- Many individuals treat fire ant bites with dilute ammonia applied topically to the affected area

TICKS

- Attach or burrow under the skin
- Flaccid paralysis can occur from neurotoxin
- Can carry organisms responsible for
  - Rocky Mountain spotted fever
    - Symptoms two to five days after tick bite
    - Fever, chills, headache, photophobia, muscle and joint pain
    - Characteristic skin rash initially on ankles and wrists, spreads to trunk, palms of hands, and soles of feet
  - Lyme disease
    - Symptoms 4 days to 22 weeks after tick bite
    - Characteristic skin rash begins as small red spot and develops into reddish circles resembling a "bull's eye"
    - Headache, fatigue, myalgias

Table 22–1. Tetanus Immunization

	Vaccine	Dosage	Age of Immunization
Child	DPT	0.5 mL	Age 2 mo, 4 mo, 6 mo, 18 mo, 4–6 yrs
Adult	Td	0.5 mL	If >5–10 yrs (depends on severity and type of wound)
	TIG	250 units	Recommended for major, unclean wounds when tetanus immunization status is unknown

DPT = diphtheria, pertussis, and tetanus; Td = tetanus and diphtheria toxoid; TIG = tetanus immunoglobulin

TETANUS PROPHYLAXIS
(see Table 22–1)

Bibliography

Budassi Sheehy S: Emergency Nursing Principles and Practice, 3rd ed. St. Louis, Mosby–Year Book, 1992.

Emergency Nurses Association: Emergency Nursing Core Curriculum, 4th ed. Philadelphia, WB Saunders, 1994.

Selfridge-Thomas J: Manual of Emergency Nursing. Philadelphia, WB Saunders, 1995.

Skidmore-Roth L: Nursing Drug Reference. St. Louis, Mosby–Year Book, 1993.

Subcommittee on Pharmacy and Therapeutics: The U. of C. Hospitals Formulary. Chicago, University of Chicago, 1995.

Chapter 23

Toxicologic Emergencies

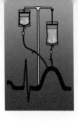

- This chapter lists common toxicologic emergencies, but it is not an exhaustive overview.
- For complete, current information on specific toxicologic emergencies, contact a local poison control center.

TOXICOLOGIC EMERGENCIES

- May be intentional or accidental
- Exposure may be by inhalation, dermal, ocular, ingestion, or parenteral routes (see Table 23–1)
- Components of the history include
  - Type and amount of substance
  - Route
  - Time of exposure
  - Treatment given prior to arrival in the ED
- Therapy is directed toward ABCs, elimination of toxin, and prevention of further absorption

ACETAMINOPHEN POISONING

- Found in many over-the-counter (OTC) preparations
- May cause delayed hepatic toxicity

Clinical Effects of Acetaminophen Poisoning

- Three phases
- Phase I: within first few hours:

Table 23–1. Toxic Syndromes

Syndrome	Manifestations	Common Causes
Narcotic	CNS depression, miosis, hypotension, hypoventilation	Narcotics, sedatives, diphenoxylate with atropine (Lomotil), propoxyphene, benzodiazepines, methaqualone, glutethemide, and pentazocine
Cholinergic	Salivation, urination, lacrimation, defecation, gastrointestinal cramping, emesis, miosis	Organophosphate and carbamate insecticides, physostigmine, neostigmine
Anticholinergic	Confusion, incoordination, hallucinations, delirium, dry skin and mucous membranes, tachycardia, mydriasis, fever, urinary retention, decreased bowel sounds	Belladonna alkaloids, certain mushrooms, antihistamines, tricyclic antidepressants, over-the-counter sleep medications, scopolamine, jimsonweed
Sympathomimetic	CNS excitation, tachycardia, seizures, hypertension	Over-the-counter cough and cold preparations, (phenylpropanolamine), theophylline, caffeine, LSD, PCP, amphetamines

Printed with permission from Wruk K, Montanio C: Toxicological emergencies. *In* Emergency Nurses Association: Emergency Nursing Core Curriculum, 4th ed. Philadelphia, WB Saunders, 1994.

- Vomiting
- Malaise
- Anorexia
- Pallor
- Phase II: next 48 hours
  - Typically asymptomatic
  - May have mild GI symptoms
  - May have mild right upper quadrant tenderness
  - Decreased urinary output
- Phase III: 3–5 days
  - Acute hepatic necrosis
  - Renal failure
  - Jaundice
  - Right upper quadrant pain
  - Hepatomegaly
  - Encephalopathy
  - Myocardiopathy

Treatment for Acetaminophen Poisoning

- ABCs
- Gastric emptying by lavage
- Do not delay charcoal administration, regardless if N-acetylcysteine (NAC) is being considered.
- Charcoal does not significantly decrease effect of NAC
- Consider toxic: ingestion of more than 7.5 gm (adult) or more than 150 mg/kg (child)
- Antidote: NAC for toxic ingestion (see Fig. 23–1)
- Initial dose = 140 mg/kg by mouth
- Dilute 10–20% solution to 5% with juice or soda to mask taste
- Subsequent doses = 70 mg/kg every 4 hours for 72 hours
- IV NAC may be considered for the patient with

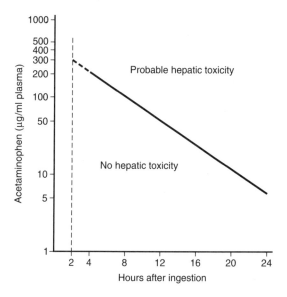

Figure 23–1. Semilogarithmic plot of plasma acetaminophen levels versus time. (From Rumak BH, Matthew H: Acetaminophen poisoning and toxicity. Pediatrics 55:871–876, 1975. Reproduced by permission of Pediatrics.)

persistent vomiting not controlled by antiemetics (Call Rocky Mountain Poison Center 1–800–525–6115 for administration information)
• Monitor liver function tests

ACID AND ALKALI INGESTION

• Acids cause severe burns to the GI tract and coagulation necrosis

- Alkalis may cause tissue necrosis within one second of exposure

Clinical Effects of Acid and Alkali Ingestion

- Alkali esophageal burns
  - Phase I: 1–2 days (inflammatory phase); perforation may occur
  - Phase II: 24–48 hours after ingestion (necrotic phase); sloughing of tissue
  - Phase III: 2–6 weeks after ingestion (constriction phase); narrowing of esophagus
- Coffee-ground emesis
- Dysphagia, drooling, chest discomfort
- Oral or pharyngeal burns
- Respiratory distress may develop because of soft tissue swelling of upper airway
- Esophageal perforation may result in mediastinitis and shock

Treatment for Acid and Alkali Ingestion

- ABCs
- Flush lips, mouth with copious amounts of water
- Dilute with milk (may use water if milk is not available)
- For significant ingestion:
  - CBC, type and crossmatch, arterial blood gases (ABGs)
  - Cardiac monitor, pulse oximetry
  - Lateral neck, chest, abdominal x-rays
- Esophagoscopy is performed within 12–24 hours after alkali ingestion
- Do not induce vomiting; lavage or give charcoal

Considerations for Acid and Alkali Ingestion

- Absence of oropharyngeal burns does not exclude esophageal injury
- Dilution of ingested material is contraindicated if perforation, shock, or respiratory distress is present
- Call the National Button Battery Ingestion Hotline 202–625–3333 in Washington, DC, for information on chemical content of batteries and clinical management recommendations

BACTERIAL FOOD POISONING

- Most common contaminants are from improper refrigeration:
  - *Staphylococcus*
  - *Salmonella*
  - *Streptococcus*
- *Clostridium* contamination associated with foods heated and kept warm more than 4 hours
- *Shigella* contamination is from human feces

Clinical Effects of Bacterial Food Poisoning

- Characteristic diarrhea: loose, watery, variable blood
- Associated symptoms:
  - Fever
  - Nausea
  - Vomiting
  - Crampy abdominal pain
  - Seizures may occur with *Shigella*
- Onset of symptoms

- *Staphylococcus* = 12–16 hours
- *Clostridium* = 12–24 hours, usually improved in 24–48 hours

Treatment for Bacterial Food Poisoning

- ABCs
- Fluid and electrolyte replacement
- Antibiotics
- Antiemetics
- Monitor serum electrolytes

BARBITURATE POISONING

- CNS depressants
- Toxicity is enhanced by alcohol and depressants
- Barbiturates include
  - Phenobarbital: long acting
  - Amobarbital, butabarbital: intermediate acting
  - Pentobarbital, secobarbital: short acting
  - Thiopental: ultra-short acting

Clinical Effects of Barbiturate Poisoning

- Altered level of consciousness, coma
- Slurred speech
- Ataxia
- Hypotension
- Respiratory arrest
- Bullae over pressure points (barbiturate burns)
- Pupillary constriction
- Hyporeflexia
- Disconjugate eye movements
- Hypothermia

Treatment for Barbiturate Poisoning

- ABCs
- Gastric lavage (emesis contraindicated because of possible rapid decrease in level of consciousness)
- Administration of charcoal and cathartic
  - First dose of charcoal and cathartic
  - Repeated doses of charcoal alone is recommended to enhance elimination and shorten the half-life of phenobarbital
- Alkalinization of urine or hemodialysis is only effective for phenobarbital

BOTULISM

- Associated with ingestion of home-preserved vegetables, fruit, or fish
- Occasionally, commercially canned foods may be the source
- Infantile botulism is associated with ingestion of honey by children less than 1 year old
- Organism: *Clostridium botulinum*

Clinical Effects of Botulism

- Onset of symptoms 12–36 hours after ingestion; may be delayed up to 4 days
- GI: nausea, vomiting
- Decreased deep tendon reflexes (DTRs)
- Dysphagia
- Dry mouth
- Sore throat
- Ptosis
- Mydriasis (dilation of pupils)
- Nystagmus

- Diplopia
- Paresis of extraocular movements (EOMs)
- Descending weakness or paralysis

Treatment for Botulism

- ABCs
- Fluid and electrolyte replacement
- Serum analysis for toxin
- Administration of antitoxin
- Consider cathartics (absorption of toxin is slow, so cathartics may be administered several hours after ingestion)

Considerations for Botulism

- Respiratory paralysis may require tracheostomy and ventilatory assistance
- May mimic stroke, Guillain-Barré syndrome, myasthenia gravis, or arsenic intoxication

CARBON MONOXIDE (CO) POISONING

- Commonly affects more than one person (family)
- Due to poor ventilation of stove, furnace, automobile exhaust, smoldering charcoal, canned heat, and wood fires
- CO is a colorless, odorless gas
- CO binds with hemoglobin at the expense of oxygen, resulting in tissue hypoxia

Clinical Effects for CO Poisoning

- Chronic exposure: recurring headaches, dizziness, nausea that is severe upon awakening and improves after leaving the home

Table 23-2. Manifestations and Treatment for Heavy Metal Poisoning

Arsenic	Lead	Mercury
	Signs and Symptoms	
Garlicky breath	Weakness, irritability, ataxia	Stomatitis
Profuse rice-like diarrhea	Weight loss	Colitis
Polyneuropathy	Personality changes	Ataxia
Abnormal KUB	Severe abdominal pain	Gingivitis
Vomiting and abdominal pain	Milky vomiting	Nephrotic syndrome
Dysrhythmias	Hypertension	
Cutaneous abnormalities	Peripheral neuropathy	
	Chelation and Metal-Specific Therapies	
Dimercaprol (BAL)	BAL	Penicillamine
Penicillamine	Penicillamine	BAL
Urine alkalinization	EDTA	Hemodialysis
Hemodialysis	Treat cerebral edema with	Treat seizures
Exchange transfusion	mannitol,	
	dexamethasone	
	Treat seizures	

- Vomiting or hematemesis
- Diarrhea
- Abdominal pain
- Latent period (6–24 hrs after ingestion)
- Systemic symptoms (4–40 hrs after ingestion)
  - Acidosis
  - Cyanosis
  - Fever
  - Shock
- Liver and renal failure (2–4 days after ingestion)
- Late complications (2–8 wks): GI obstruction

Treatment for Iron Toxicity

- ABCs
- Prevent absorption of iron
  - Lavage
  - Ipecac syrup within first 30 minutes after ingestion
- Chelation therapy with deferoxamine mesylate:
  - Chelation agent = any compound, usually organic, that has 2 or more points of attachment at which an atom of metal may be joined to form a ring-type structure
  - If serum iron level is unavailable, and the patient is symptomatic, deferoxamine dose = 90 mg/kg/dose IM and repeat every 8 hours

Considerations for Iron Toxicity

- A change in urine color from pink to orange-red indicates a positive response to chelation therapy
- X-ray will detect undissolved iron tablets in the stomach
- 60 mg/kg iron is a lethal dose

ORGANOPHOSPHATE POISONING

- Inhibits acetylcholinesterase
- Absorption is through skin and GI routes
- Produces classic cholinergic syndrome

Clinical Effects of Organophosphate Poisoning

- SLUDGE mnemonic is indicative of muscarinic symptoms
  - S = **S**alivation
  - L = **L**acrimation
  - U = **U**rination
  - D = **D**efecation
  - G = **G**I cramping
  - E = **E**mesis
- Nicotinic symptoms include motor findings:
  - Muscle cramps
  - Weakness
  - Hyperreflexia
  - Fasciculations
- CNS symptoms include
  - Restlessness
  - Ataxia
  - Confusion
  - Coma

Treatment for Organophosphate Poisoning

- ABCs
  - Decontamination of skin
  - Prevent absorption
  - Lavage (do not induce vomiting)

- Activated charcoal with sorbitol
- Atropine (binds at muscarinic receptors): 0.05 mg/kg/dose up to 2–5 mg/dose
- Pralidoxime (2-PAM) (reactivates acetylcholinesterase and reverses cholinergic nicotinic stimulation)
  - Given after atropinization
  - Useful if given within 36 hours of exposure
  - 20 mg/kg/dose up to 2 gm/dose IV slowly
- Considerations: expect tachycardia because of atropinization

PETROLEUM DISTILLATE/ HYDROCARBON EXPOSURE

- Absorbed through GI and skin routes
- Aspiration is a serious problem
- Common ingredient:
  - Kerosene
  - Gasoline
  - Naphthalene (mothballs)
  - Furniture polish and oils
  - Paint thinner
  - Lighter fluid
  - Turpentine
  - Motor oil
  - Camphor
- High viscosity = limited or low toxicity
- Low viscosity = high toxicity due to possible aspiration

Clinical Effects of Petroleum Distillate/Hydrocarbon Exposure

- Cutaneous (eczematoid dermatitis to full-thickness burns)

- GI (burns to oropharynx, nausea, vomiting, abdominal pain, and diarrhea)
- Pulmonary (cyanosis, bronchospasm, wheezing, intercostal and subcostal retractions, hemoptysis, pulmonary edema, fever)
- CNS (suppression of ventilatory drive, headache, ataxia, blurred vision, dizziness, lethargy, stupor, coma)
- Cardiac (cardiomyopathy, ventricular tachycardia, myocardial injury)

Treatment for Petroleum Distillate/Hydrocarbon Exposure

- ABCs
- Supplemental oxygen
- Skin decontamination
- Prevent absorption: GI lavage is not indicated unless a large ingestion
- Treat the symptoms

- CHAMP mnemonic for toxic additives:
  - C = **C**amphor
  - H = **H**alogenated hydrocarbons (carbon tetrachloride)
  - A = **A**romatic benzenes
  - M = **M**etals
  - P = **P**esticides

- Considerations: One swallow in a child = approximately 4 mL

PLANT POISONING

- Many forms of toxic plants are common, often decorative foliage or fruits.

- Common poisonous plants include (but are not limited to)
  - Bird of paradise: pods and seeds
  - Dumbcane: especially the stem and leaves
  - Elephant's ears: especially the stem and leaves
  - English ivy: especially the leaves and berries
  - Foxglove
  - Holly: berries and leaves
  - Lily of the Valley: all parts
  - Mistletoe: berries
  - Poinsettia: all parts
  - Rhubarb: leaf blades
  - Peach pits
  - Cherry pits
  - Apricot pits
  - Plum pits
  - Pear seeds
  - Certain mushrooms
- Ingestion is the entry route

Clinical Effects of Plant Poisoning

- Oral burning, numbness or pain
- GI disturbances
- CNS (altered mental status)

Treatment for Plant Poisoning

- Dependent upon the substance
- ABCs
- GI lavage
- Antihistamines
- Treat the symptoms
- Respiratory support
- Digoxin immune Fab (Digibind)

- Pain control
- Atropine
- Considerations: Consult your local Poison Control Center for identification and appropriate treatment

SALICYLATE POISONING

- GI absorption through ingestion (see Fig. 23–2)
- Common ingredient in over-the-counter (OTC) preparations

Clinical Effects of Salicylate Poisoning

- Tinnitus
- GI disturbances
- Renal failure
- Tachypnea
- Mental status changes
  - Lethargy
  - Excitability
  - Seizures
  - Coma
- Slurred speech
- Hallucinations
- Systemic collapse
- Allergic reactions

Treatment for Salicylate Poisoning

- ABCs
- Prevent absorption
  - Gastric lavage
  - Activated charcoal with sorbitol (use sorbitol with caution in children)
- Alkalinization of urine pH to 7–8

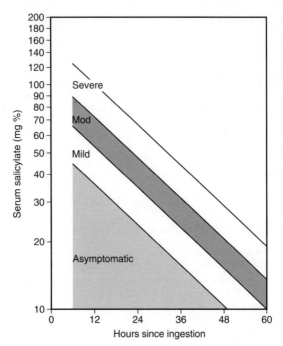

Figure 23–2. Nomogram relating serum salicylate concentration and expected severity of intoxication at varying intervals following the ingestion of a single dose of salicylate. (From Done AK: Salicylate intoxication. Pediatrics 26:805, 1960. Reproduced by permission of Pediatrics.)

- Treat any seizures
- Dialysis for renal failure
- Considerations: a quantitative test for presence of aspirin in urine: add a few drops of 10% ferric chloride to 5 mL of urine (if aspirin is present, the urine will turn purple)

SEDATIVES AND HYPNOTIC POISONING

- CNS depressants
- Potentiated by alcohol or depressants
- Commonly prescribed drugs
  - Benzodiazepines
    - Alprazolam (Xanax)
    - Lorazepam (Ativan)
    - Diazepam (Valium)
  - Alcohol (common additive to cough preparations)
  - Meprobamate (Equanil, Miltown, Kalmm)
  - Glutethimide (Doriden, Rolathimide)
  - Methaqualone (Quaalude)

Clinical Effects of Sedatives or Hypnotic Poisoning

- Altered mental status (stupor, coma, seizures)
- Cardiovascular disturbances
  - Arrhythmias
  - Hypotension
- Respiratory depression
- GI disturbances

Treatment for Sedatives or Hypnotic Poisoning

- ABCs
- Prevent absorption
  - Lavage
  - Activated charcoal with sorbitol
  - Do not induce vomiting because of rapid onset of CNS side effects
- Flumazenil (Romazicon) is a benzodiazepine receptor antagonist

269

- Adult dose: 0.2 mg (2 mL) given over 30 seconds, wait 30 seconds, then give 0.3 mg; if consciousness does not occur may give 0.5 mg (5 mL) at 60-second intervals up to a maximum dose of 3 mg
- Considerations: Benzodiazepines are the most commonly abused sedative but least likely to cause respiratory depression when used alone (i.e., no other depressants or alcohol)

TRICYCLIC ANTIDEPRESSANT POISONING

- Commonly prescribed for antidepressant therapy and also bedwetting treatment
- Amitriptyline HCl: Amitril, Elavil, Emitrip, Endep, Enovil
- Doxepin HCl: Adapin, Sinequan
- Imipramine HCl: Tofranil, Vanimine, Ropramine, Tipramine
- Amoxapine: Asendin
- Desipramine HCl: Norpramin, Pertofrane
- Nortriptyline HCl: Aventyl, Pamelor
- The major toxicity is from anticholinergic and quinidine-like effects

Clinical Effects of Tricyclic Antidepressant Poisoning

- Dry, flushed skin
- Dilated pupils
- Urinary retention
- Dysrythmias due to cardiotoxicity
- Altered level of consciousness
- Seizures
- Coma
- Hypotension (common)

Treatment for Tricyclic Antidepressant Poisoning

- ABCs
- EKG
- Pulse oximetry
- Prevent absorption
  - Lavage
  - Activated charcoal with sorbitol
  - Do not induce vomiting due to rapid deterioration and possible loss of airway
- Use physostigmine with extreme caution
- Respiratory support
- Considerations: deterioration is very rapid, expect to intubate as needed

ACTIVATED CHARCOAL TIPS

- Dosages:
  - Adults: 1 gm/kg; 50–100 gm
  - Children: 1 gm/kg; 15–50 gm
- Activated charcoal is given after lavage or emesis, or alone if ingestion occurred more than 1 hour before arrival in the ED
- May administer orally or via nasogastric/ orogastric tube
- Charcoal can sometimes stain clothing and shoes. Wear personal protective equipment

ACTIVATED CHARCOAL WITH SORBITOL

- Dosages:
  - Adults: 1 gm/kg activated charcoal in 70% sorbitol
  - Children: 1 gm/kg activated charcoal mixed in

35–70% sorbitol in children more than 1 year of age
- Given as an initial dose only; subsequent doses of activated charcoal are *without* sorbitol
- Multiple-dose activated charcoal
  - Adults: 20–50 gm every 4–6 hours
  - Children: 0.5 gm/kg/dose every 4–6 hours

Bibliography

Barkin RM, Rosen P: Emergency Pediatrics, 4th ed. St. Louis, Mosby–Year Book, 1994.

Budassi Sheehy S: Manual of Emergency Care, 3rd ed. St. Louis, CV Mosby, 1990.

Emergency Nurses Association: Emergency Nursing Core Curriculum, 4th ed. Philadelphia, WB Saunders, 1994.

Fischbach F: A Manual of Laboratory Diagnostic Tests. Philadelphia, JB Lippincott, 1980.

Goldfrank L, Flomenbaum N, Lewin N, et al: Goldfrank's Toxicologic Emergencies, 5th ed. Norwalk, Appleton & Lange, 1994.

Kitt S, Selfridge-Thomas J, Proehl J, Kaiser J: Emergency Nursing: A Physiologic and Clinical Perspective, 2nd ed. Philadelphia, WB Saunders, 1995.

Chapter 24
Transfer and Transport

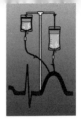

PREPARATION OF THE PATIENT FOR TRANSPORT

Transferring Hospital Responsibilities

- Activate the transfer process. Physicians must obtain approval from another physician willing to accept the patient at the receiving facility
- Ascertain if the receiving facility has qualified personnel and adequate space to provide the level of care required
- Perform treatments and diagnostic studies requested by the receiving facility
- Assure appropriate personnel and equipment are present during transport
- ***Resuscitation and stabilization of the patient is simultaneous with the transfer process***

Nursing Interventions

- Secure and maintain a patent airway
- Maintain full spinal immobilization (if indicated)
- Ensure adequate breathing
- Ensure adequate circulation
- Insert a gastric tube (if indicated)
- Insert urinary catheter (if indicated)
- Splint any suspected fractures

- Monitor cardiac rhythm and rate, blood pressure, respiratory rate, pulse oximetry, intake and output
- Administer medications as prescribed:
  - Methylprednisolone for spinal cord injury (see Chapter 14)
  - Tetanus prophylaxis as indicated (see Chapter 22)
  - Antibiotics
  - Analgesics
  - Antianxiety agents (as indicated)
- Obtain consent for transfer
- Copy the clinical record, radiographic studies, laboratory results, and advanced directives
- Allow the family or significant other(s) to see the patient
- Document a list of patient's valuables and disposition of valuables
- Provide written directions and maps to family. Advise family to use caution and obey traffic laws.
- Give nurse-to-nurse report to the receiving hospital
- Document actual date and time of transfer

AIRCRAFT SAFETY RULES

- The ultimate responsibility rests with the pilot for safe operation of the aircraft.
- Safety rules include
  - Never shine lights toward the aircraft on landing and takeoff
  - Secure small pieces of equipment and loose articles before approaching an aircraft
  - Keep the landing zone clear of trees, wires, and other obstacles (rotor wing). Landing zone minimum space is 100×100 feet.

- Do not mark landing zone with loose articles
- Do not allow people or equipment within a minimum of 100 feet of the landing perimeter
- Do not approach the aircraft until signalled by a crew member
- When approaching the aircraft, do so in full view of the pilot
- Approach rotor-wing aircraft from downhill side only and never from the rear
- Allow the flight crew to direct loading and unloading of equipment and patient(s).

Bibliography

Taskforce on Interhospital Transport, American Academy of Pediatrics: Guidelines for Air and Ground Transport of Neonatal and Pediatric Patients. Elk Grove Village, IL, American Academy of Pediatrics, 1993.

Emergency Nurses Association: Trauma Nursing Core Course Instructor Manual, 4th ed. Park Ridge, IL, ENA, 1995.

Chapter 25
Triage

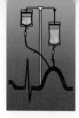

URGENCY RATINGS

- A systematic classification of patients based on severity of illness or injury
- May include three, four, or five urgency levels
- Three-level urgency ratings are the most common and easiest to use

Emergent Rating

CRITERIA

- Immediate threat to life, limb, or vision
- Requires immediate medical attention

EXAMPLES OF EMERGENT RATING

- Cardiopulmonary arrest
- Respiratory distress
- Major burns
- Multi-system trauma, major trauma
- Anaphylaxis
- Active seizure
- Coma
- Neurovascular compromise
- Uncontrolled bleeding
- Fever in an infant less than two months of age
- Cardiac chest pain

Urgent Rating

CRITERIA

- Requires prompt treatment, within two hours
- Stable vital signs

EXAMPLES OF URGENT RATING

- Lacerations, bleeding controlled
- Nondisplaced fractures; no neurovascular impairment
- Febrile seizure, child alert
- Asthma, no respiratory distress
- Moderate burns
- Abdominal pain
- Noncardiac chest pain
- Fever
- Patients with nonurgent presenting complaints with significant chronic illness

Nonurgent Rating

CRITERIA

- Minor illness or injury
- Treatment required, time is not a factor
- Patients often seek care in the ED for routine medical care (no primary care provider or primary care provider is not available)

EXAMPLES OF NONURGENT RATING

- Sore throat
- Minor sprains, strains
- Rashes
- Minor upper respiratory infection (URI) or flu symptoms

- Prescription refills
- Constipation
- Vaginal discharge
- Return to work or school notes

TRIAGE ASSESSMENT

- Obtain a chief complaint in the patient's own words
- Use open-ended questions
- Document a subjective and objective assessment
- Determine urgency rating: Facilitate placement of patients with "emergent" rating without delay
- Implement treatment or diagnostic procedures, which may include
  - Application of cold packs, elevation, and splinting for musculoskeletal injuries
  - Administration of antipyretics
  - Collection of urine specimen in suspected UTI
  - Application of direct pressure to control bleeding
  - Minor wound asepsis and application of dressings
  - Urine pregnancy testing
- Facilitate placement in appropriate patient care area
- Re-evaluate patients remaining in waiting area according to urgency rating, changes in condition, and departmental policy.

TRIAGE GUIDELINES

- Always begin with the primary assessment ABCs
- Many guidelines and mnemonics exist to facilitate obtaining a complete triage assessment

TRIAGE MNEMONICS

- OLD CART
  - O = **O**nset of symptoms
  - L = **L**ocation of problem
  - D = **D**uration of symptoms
  - C = **C**haracteristics of the symptoms described by the patient
  - A = **A**ggravating factors
  - R = **R**elieving factors
  - T = **T**reatment administered before arrival

- PQRST format, useful with a chief complaint of "pain"
  - P = **P**rovokes
  - Q = **Q**uality
  - R = **R**adiation
  - S = **S**everity (use a rating scale)
  - T = **T**iming

- SAVE A CHILD
  - For recognition of a seriously ill pediatric patient (courtesy of Emergency Nurses Association, State Council, Hawaii)
  - SAVE: observations made prior to touching the child
  - CHILD: history from caretaker and brief examination
    - S = **S**kin: mottled, cyanotic, petechiae, pallor?
    - A = **A**ctivity: needs assistance? not ambulatory? responsive?
    - V = **V**entilation: retractions? head bobbing? drooling? nasal flaring? slow rate? fast rate? stridor? wheezing?
    - E = **E**ye contact: glassy stare? fails to engage/focus?
    - A = **A**buse: unexplained bruising/injuries? inappropriate parent?
    - C = **C**ry: high pitched cephalic? irritable?
    - H = **H**eat: high fever greater than 41°C? hypothermia less than 36°C?
    - I = **I**mmune System: sickle cell? AIDS? corticosteroids?
    - L = **L**evel of consciousness: irritable? lethargic? pain only? convulsing? unresponsive?
    - D = **D**ehydration: hollow eyes? capillary refill? cold hands, feet? voiding? severe diarrhea? vomiting: projectile, bilious persistent? dry mucous membranes?

CIAMPEDs (see Table 25-1)

Table 25-1. CIAMPEDS: Triage History

Format	Questions
C = Chief complaint	*Why was the child brought to the emergency department? What is the primary problem/concern and duration of complaint?*
I = Immunizations	*Are they up to date? When were they last given?*
= Isolation	*Has the child recently been exposed to any communicable diseases?*
A = Allergies	*Does the child have any known allergies? Is the child allergic to any medications? What was the child's reaction to the medication?*
M = Medications	*Is the child taking any prescription drugs or over-the-counter drugs (e.g., acetaminophen)? When was the last dose administered and how much was given? Is the child on immunosuppressive medications?*
P = Past medical history	*Does the child have a history of any significant illness, injury, or hospitalization? Does the child have a known chronic illness?*
Parents' impression of child's condition	*What is different about the child's condition that concerns the caregiver?*
E = Events surrounding the illness or injury	*How long has the child been ill? Was the onset rapid or slow? Has anyone else in the family been ill? If the emergency visit is for an injury, when did the injury occur, was it witnessed, and what happened?*
D = Diet	*How much has the child been eating and drinking? When was the last time the child ate or drank?*

From Emergency Nurses Association: Emergency Nursing Pediatric Course Park Ridge, IL, ENA, 1993.

Bibliography

Donatelli N (ed): Emergency Nurses Association Standards of Emergency Nursing Practice, 3rd ed. St. Louis, Mosby–Year Book, 1995.

Emergency Nurses Association: Emergency Nursing Core Curriculum, 4th ed. Philadelphia, WB Saunders, 1994.

Emergency Nurses Association: Emergency Nursing Pediatric Course Instructor Manual. 1st ed. Park Ridge, IL, Emergency Nurses Association, 1993.

Emergency Nurses Association: Triage: Meeting the Challenge. Park Ridge, IL, Emergency Nurses Association, 1992.

Kitt S, Selfridge-Thomas J, Proehl J, Kaiser J: Emergency Nursing: A Physiologic and Clinical Perspective, 2nd ed. Philadelphia, WB Saunders, 1995.

Sullivan R: Triage: A subspecialty of emergency nursing. Emphasis: Nursing: 26–33, 1989.

Index

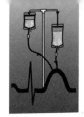

Note: Page numbers in *italics* refer to illustrations; page numbers followed by t refer to tables.